Chapter 1: Understanding the Vagus Nerve

The vagus nerve is often referred to as the "wandering nerve" because of its far-reaching influence throughout the body. It plays a pivotal role in regulating many of our body's functions, many of which we don't consciously control. But how exactly does this nerve work, and why is it so important for our overall well-being?

Anatomy of the Vagus Nerve

The vagus nerve is the tenth cranial nerve, and it extends from the brainstem down to various organs in the chest and abdomen. It is the longest nerve in the autonomic nervous system (ANS), which controls involuntary bodily functions. The vagus nerve originates in the brainstem, specifically from the medulla oblongata, and it travels down through the neck, chest, and abdomen, innervating vital organs such as the heart, lungs, and digestive system.

This nerve is a part of the parasympathetic nervous system (PNS), which is responsible for the body's "rest and digest" activities. The vagus nerve controls several physiological processes such as heart rate, digestion, respiratory rate, and even aspects of mood regulation. Its far-reaching network makes it an essential component in the maintenance of homeostasis in the body.

The Role of the Vagus Nerve in the Body

The vagus nerve performs multiple functions essential for maintaining internal balance, otherwise known as homeostasis. It helps to manage the body's stress response, regulate inflammation, control heart rate, promote digestion, and even communicate with the brain to influence emotional states. It is deeply involved in the regulation of the autonomic nervous system, which balances the body's automatic functions without requiring conscious effort.

At its core, the vagus nerve helps the body transition from a state of stress (sympathetic response) to one of rest and recovery (parasympathetic response). When it is activated, it promotes a state of relaxation, reduces heart rate, and enhances digestion, enabling the body to recuperate and restore energy.

In this way, the vagus nerve is an essential player in maintaining balance, or "equilibrium," within the body and mind. It ensures that we are able to respond to stress effectively, while also allowing us to recover and recharge when necessary.

Vagus Nerve and the Autonomic Nervous System

The autonomic nervous system (ANS) is responsible for regulating many unconscious functions that keep us alive, such as breathing, heartbeat, and digestion. The ANS is divided into two main branches: the sympathetic nervous system and the parasympathetic nervous system. The vagus nerve is the primary nerve of the parasympathetic branch.

While the sympathetic nervous system is activated during periods of stress or danger, triggering the "fight or flight" response, the parasympathetic nervous system is responsible for returning the body to a relaxed state. The vagus nerve plays a vital role in this process by initiating the "rest and digest" functions. When the vagus nerve is stimulated, it calms the body down, reduces heart rate, and triggers processes that allow the body to heal and restore itself.

Key Functions: Parasympathetic Control

One of the most important roles of the vagus nerve is its parasympathetic control over several bodily functions. Here are some of the key functions it helps regulate:

1. **Heart Rate**: The vagus nerve works to slow down the heart rate in response to stress or physical activity. This effect is known as "vagal tone." Higher vagal tone is associated with better cardiovascular health, while lower vagal tone is linked to heart disease and other conditions.
2. **Breathing**: The vagus nerve influences breathing rate by controlling the muscles that regulate respiratory function. It slows the breathing rate, aiding relaxation and reducing stress.
3. **Digestion**: The vagus nerve has a crucial role in digestion by stimulating the release of digestive enzymes and controlling gut motility. It also helps regulate the gut-brain axis, a vital communication network between the digestive system and the brain.
4. **Inflammation**: The vagus nerve has an anti-inflammatory effect on the body. It can reduce the production of pro-inflammatory cytokines and help regulate immune function, making it vital in managing chronic inflammation and autoimmune disorders.
5. **Mood and Stress**: The vagus nerve has been shown to influence emotional regulation. By activating the parasympathetic response, it reduces the production of stress hormones such as cortisol and promotes feelings of calmness and well-being.

Vagal Tone and Its Importance

When we talk about the vagus nerve, we often refer to "vagal tone." This term refers to the level of activity in the vagus nerve and its effect on the body's functions. A high vagal tone is associated with resilience to stress, better mental health, and improved physical health. Conversely, a low vagal tone is linked to a variety of conditions, including anxiety, depression, cardiovascular problems, and autoimmune diseases.

Vagal tone can be measured by looking at heart rate variability (HRV), a metric that tracks the fluctuations in time between heartbeats. A high HRV indicates a strong vagal tone, which is associated with better stress resilience, emotional regulation, and overall health.

In the chapters ahead, we will explore how to enhance vagal tone through various practices, from breathing exercises and meditation to physical exercise and nutrition. Mastering your vagus nerve and optimizing its function can lead to profound improvements in both mental and physical health.

The Vagus Nerve's Connection to the Gut–Brain Axis

An important aspect of the vagus nerve's function is its relationship with the gut-brain axis. This communication network links the central nervous system (CNS) with the enteric nervous system (ENS), which controls the digestive system. The vagus nerve acts as a two-way communication channel between the brain and the gut.

Recent research has highlighted the critical role of the vagus nerve in gut health, revealing how it can influence digestion, immune response, and even mood. For example, when the vagus nerve is stimulated, it can improve digestion and help reduce symptoms of gastrointestinal disorders like irritable bowel syndrome (IBS) and inflammatory bowel disease (IBD).

Moreover, the gut-brain axis is crucial for emotional regulation. The gut produces a large amount of serotonin, a neurotransmitter that regulates mood, and much of this serotonin is communicated to the brain via the vagus nerve. This has led scientists to recognize the vagus nerve as a potential therapeutic target for treating mental health conditions like depression and anxiety.

Conclusion

The vagus nerve is a vital and versatile component of our nervous system, influencing a vast array of bodily functions, from heart rate and digestion to mood and stress response. In this chapter, we've explored the anatomy of the vagus nerve, its role in the body, and its connection to the autonomic nervous system. Understanding its functions is the first step toward mastering it and unlocking the potential it holds for improving our health and well-being.

In the next chapter, we will dive deeper into the science of the vagus nerve, exploring how it communicates with the body and the brain, and how its activation can transform our physical and mental health.

Chapter 2: The Science of the Vagus Nerve

In Chapter 1, we introduced the vagus nerve as an essential component of the body's autonomic nervous system. We explored its anatomy, its role in regulating critical bodily functions, and its deep connection to the parasympathetic system. In this chapter, we will delve deeper into the scientific mechanisms that enable the vagus nerve to influence and communicate with various systems in the body, as well as how it maintains balance and harmony within us.

Signals and Pathways: How the Vagus Nerve Communicates

The vagus nerve is often described as the body's "communication highway" because it transmits signals between the brain and numerous organs. To truly appreciate the power of the vagus nerve, it's essential to understand the pathways through which these signals travel.

The vagus nerve communicates via both sensory (afferent) and motor (efferent) pathways. Sensory pathways carry information from the organs back to the brain, including feedback about heart rate, gut activity, and even blood pressure. This allows the brain to constantly monitor the body's internal environment and adjust accordingly. The motor pathways, on the other hand, send signals from the brain to the organs to initiate actions like slowing the heart rate or increasing digestive enzyme production.

One of the most fascinating aspects of the vagus nerve is its ability to integrate both sensory and motor information in real time. This two-way communication allows for precise regulation of many physiological processes, from controlling the heartbeat to managing inflammation. The vagus nerve is constantly monitoring the body's condition and making adjustments to keep things in balance.

Neural Pathways and Brain Connectivity

The vagus nerve is intricately connected to several important areas of the brain, which contribute to its ability to regulate bodily functions. The vagus nerve originates in the brainstem, a critical region that acts as the brain's command center for regulating involuntary functions. From there, it projects throughout the body, connecting with the heart, lungs, digestive organs, and other vital systems.

One of the key areas where the vagus nerve exerts its influence is the **medulla oblongata**, part of the brainstem that controls critical functions such as breathing, heart rate, and blood pressure. Through this connection, the vagus nerve is able to regulate these functions automatically, ensuring they remain within healthy ranges.

Additionally, the vagus nerve plays a role in modulating the **hypothalamus** and **limbic system**, two areas involved in regulating emotional responses, stress, and memory. This connection underscores why the vagus nerve is often referred to as a key player in the mind-body connection. The vagus nerve helps bridge the gap between physical health and emotional well-being, offering a pathway to balance both.

Furthermore, recent research has shown that the vagus nerve is a key participant in a variety of higher-order cognitive functions. These include attention, decision-making, and emotional regulation. By influencing structures like the **prefrontal cortex**, which governs executive functions, the vagus nerve helps maintain cognitive performance under stress and plays a role in the modulation of mood.

The Vagus Nerve's Influence on the Gut-Brain Axis

One of the most compelling areas of vagus nerve research is its role in the **gut-brain axis**. The gut-brain axis is the bi-directional communication network that links the brain to the digestive system. The vagus nerve plays a central role in this communication, influencing digestion and emotional states alike.

Approximately 90% of the fibers in the vagus nerve are sensory fibers, which relay information from the gut to the brain. This means the vagus nerve is constantly transmitting signals that tell the brain about what is happening in the digestive system. For example, the vagus nerve provides feedback about how well food is being digested, whether the stomach is full, or whether there are any issues such as bloating or discomfort.

But the influence of the vagus nerve goes beyond simply informing the brain about digestive processes. The gut itself has a significant impact on our mental and emotional health, primarily through the production of neurotransmitters such as serotonin. In fact, the gut is often referred to as the "second brain" because it produces around 95% of the body's serotonin, a neurotransmitter that regulates mood, appetite, and sleep.

The vagus nerve, in turn, helps communicate this information to the brain. This connection underscores the importance of gut health not only for digestion but for overall emotional well-being. A healthy gut microbiome can influence vagal tone, which then affects mood, stress resilience, and even cognitive function.

Research suggests that improving vagal tone through practices like meditation, yoga, and deep breathing can help improve gut health, and vice versa. As we continue to explore the vagus nerve in the coming chapters, we will look at how this gut-brain communication influences everything from stress levels to immune function.

The Vagus Nerve and Inflammation Regulation

Another remarkable aspect of the vagus nerve is its ability to modulate inflammation in the body. Inflammation is the body's natural response to injury or infection, but when it becomes chronic, it can contribute to a wide range of health issues, including heart disease, diabetes, and autoimmune disorders. The vagus nerve plays a key role in controlling inflammation by signaling the brain to release anti-inflammatory molecules.

The vagus nerve interacts with the immune system via the **cholinergic anti-inflammatory pathway**. When activated, the vagus nerve releases acetylcholine, a neurotransmitter that binds to receptors on immune cells, reducing the production of pro-inflammatory cytokines. This mechanism helps protect the body from the harmful effects of chronic inflammation, which has been implicated in conditions such as rheumatoid arthritis, inflammatory bowel disease, and even depression.

This anti-inflammatory effect of the vagus nerve is one of the reasons why vagal stimulation has been explored as a potential treatment for conditions related to inflammation. Researchers are looking into vagus nerve stimulation (VNS) therapies for a variety of conditions, including depression, Crohn's disease, and sepsis.

The Role of the Vagus Nerve in Stress and Relaxation

The vagus nerve is central to how we respond to stress. When we are faced with a stressful situation, the body initiates a "fight-or-flight" response, a physiological reaction controlled by the sympathetic nervous system. This response increases heart rate, blood pressure, and respiration to prepare the body for action.

However, once the stressor has passed, the parasympathetic nervous system, with the vagus nerve at its helm, kicks in to restore balance. The vagus nerve helps to slow the heart rate, lower blood pressure, and initiate the relaxation response, bringing the body back to a calm and balanced state.

In chronic stress or anxiety, the vagus nerve's ability to activate the parasympathetic system may be diminished, which is why those with high levels of stress may experience difficulty relaxing or recovering from stressful events. By practicing techniques such as deep breathing or meditation, which stimulate the vagus nerve, we can enhance our ability to switch from stress to relaxation, improving overall well-being and resilience.

Conclusion

The vagus nerve is an intricate and multifaceted nerve that plays a crucial role in communication between the brain and the body. Through its extensive network of sensory and motor pathways, it helps regulate a wide array of functions, from heart rate and digestion to mood and immune response. By understanding the vagus nerve's communication pathways and its influence on both the body and brain, we can begin to appreciate its immense potential for improving health and well-being.

In the next chapter, we will explore the mind-body connection in more detail, examining how the vagus nerve influences emotional health and stress management. We'll uncover how vagal activation can help you achieve a balanced and harmonious life, both physically and mentally.

Chapter 3: The Vagus Nerve and the Mind–Body Connection

The mind and body are not separate entities; rather, they are intricately connected through a complex network of neurons, hormones, and biochemical signals. One of the key players in this communication is the vagus nerve. It not only regulates bodily functions like heart rate and digestion but also deeply influences emotional states, stress responses, and mental well-being. In this chapter, we will explore how the vagus nerve serves as the bridge between the mind and body, helping us achieve emotional balance and manage stress.

How the Vagus Nerve Affects Emotions

The vagus nerve plays a central role in emotional regulation by controlling the parasympathetic nervous system, which is often referred to as the "rest and digest" system. The parasympathetic system is responsible for calming the body after it has been activated by stress, thus helping to restore balance after a "fight or flight" response triggered by the sympathetic nervous system.

When the vagus nerve is functioning optimally, it promotes relaxation and emotional stability. It helps decrease the physical manifestations of stress, such as a rapid heartbeat or shallow breathing, by signaling the body to relax. This is why the vagus nerve is often considered a "calming" nerve—its activation brings us back to a state of peace and relaxation.

The vagus nerve's influence on the brain is also significant. It is directly connected to brain regions that regulate mood, including the limbic system, which is responsible for emotional processing and memory. The vagus nerve can help reduce feelings of anxiety, depression, and even anger by promoting a calm, regulated state of mind.

In addition, the vagus nerve plays a role in social bonding. Research has shown that when the vagus nerve is activated, it enhances social interactions by promoting positive facial expressions and a calm demeanor. This is why vagal tone—how well the vagus nerve is functioning—has been linked to the ability to connect with others and navigate social situations with ease.

Stress, Anxiety, and the Vagus Nerve

Stress is a natural part of life, but chronic stress can have serious consequences for both physical and mental health. Chronic activation of the sympathetic nervous system —our body's stress response—can lead to elevated levels of stress hormones like cortisol, which over time can weaken the immune system, contribute to cardiovascular issues, and even impair cognitive function. The vagus nerve provides an important counterbalance to this stress response by activating the parasympathetic system, which restores calm and promotes relaxation.

When the vagus nerve is not functioning optimally, the body remains stuck in a constant state of "fight or flight." This can lead to chronic anxiety, increased heart rate, shallow breathing, and digestive issues. Vagal dysfunction has been implicated in conditions such as generalized anxiety disorder, post-traumatic stress disorder (PTSD), and panic attacks.

However, the good news is that the vagus nerve is highly adaptable. Through specific exercises and techniques, we can activate the vagus nerve and reduce the effects of stress and anxiety. In fact, research has shown that regular vagal stimulation can help reduce symptoms of anxiety and improve overall mental well-being.

One of the most effective ways to activate the vagus nerve and combat stress is through **vagus nerve stimulation (VNS)**, which can be done in several ways, including through breathing exercises, mindfulness meditation, and even cold exposure. Vagus nerve stimulation has been shown to increase heart rate variability (HRV), a key indicator of the body's ability to respond to stress in a healthy way. Higher HRV is associated with better emotional regulation, resilience to stress, and improved mental health.

Balancing the Body and Mind through Vagal Activation

The relationship between the body and mind is a two-way street, and the vagus nerve is one of the primary conduits for this communication. By activating the vagus nerve, we can influence both physical and emotional well-being. In essence, when we calm the body, we also calm the mind, and vice versa.

Breathing is one of the most powerful ways to activate the vagus nerve and bring about this mind-body balance. Deep, slow breathing—especially **diaphragmatic breathing**—is highly effective in stimulating the vagus nerve and engaging the parasympathetic nervous system. By consciously slowing down our breath, we signal to our body that it is safe to relax, reducing the production of stress hormones and promoting a sense of calm.

Another way to activate the vagus nerve and improve emotional regulation is through **meditation and mindfulness practices**. These practices focus on cultivating awareness of the present moment and calming the mind. Mindfulness has been shown to increase vagal tone, which can enhance emotional resilience and improve mental health outcomes.

In addition to these practices, **social connection** plays a significant role in vagal activation. Engaging in meaningful interactions with others, whether through conversation, touch, or shared experiences, can activate the vagus nerve and promote feelings of safety and trust. This is why close relationships and a strong social network are often associated with better mental health and well-being.

Even activities that promote a sense of joy and relaxation—such as listening to music, spending time in nature, or engaging in creative expression—can stimulate the vagus nerve and contribute to a more balanced and peaceful state of mind. In fact, studies have shown that people with higher vagal tone are generally more adaptable to stress, more socially engaged, and more capable of managing difficult emotions.

Vagal Stimulation and Mental Health Disorders

Vagal tone is closely linked to mental health, and several conditions—such as depression, anxiety, PTSD, and even bipolar disorder—are associated with low vagal tone. Low vagal tone means that the body struggles to shift from a state of high alert (stress) back to a calm, balanced state, leading to chronic emotional dysregulation.

Fortunately, there are effective ways to address vagal dysfunction and improve mental health. One such approach is **vagus nerve stimulation (VNS)** therapy, which involves using electrical impulses to stimulate the vagus nerve. While VNS therapy is typically used for treatment-resistant depression and epilepsy, emerging evidence suggests it may also be beneficial for other mental health conditions.

For individuals who are not undergoing VNS therapy, there are numerous non-invasive techniques that can stimulate the vagus nerve naturally. These include **deep breathing exercises, progressive muscle relaxation**, and **yoga**. By practicing these techniques regularly, individuals can increase vagal tone, reduce symptoms of anxiety and depression, and improve overall emotional regulation.

Practical Tips for Enhancing Vagal Tone

1. **Practice deep breathing**: Engage in diaphragmatic breathing, also known as abdominal breathing, to stimulate the vagus nerve. Aim for slow, deep breaths that fill your diaphragm, rather than shallow chest breathing. Try incorporating a breathing technique such as the **4-7-8 method**—inhale for 4 seconds, hold for 7 seconds, and exhale for 8 seconds.
2. **Meditation and mindfulness**: Regular meditation practices, such as guided meditation, mindfulness, or loving-kindness meditation, can help activate the vagus nerve and promote emotional stability.
3. **Cold exposure**: Brief cold exposure, such as splashing your face with cold water or taking cold showers, can stimulate the vagus nerve and activate the parasympathetic nervous system, reducing stress.
4. **Engage in social connection**: Spend quality time with loved ones, engage in meaningful conversations, or practice positive touch, such as hugging or holding hands. Social connection is a natural way to activate the vagus nerve and improve emotional well-being.
5. **Exercise regularly**: Physical exercise, especially aerobic activities like walking, running, or swimming, can improve vagal tone and help reduce stress and anxiety.

Conclusion

The vagus nerve is a powerful tool in regulating both the body and mind. By understanding how it affects emotional states and stress responses, we can begin to harness its power to create balance and emotional well-being. In this chapter, we explored how the vagus nerve influences our emotions, regulates stress, and promotes mental health. Through specific practices like deep breathing, meditation, and social connection, we can activate the vagus nerve to enhance emotional resilience and foster a greater sense of calm.

In the next chapter, we will delve into the healing power of the vagus nerve, examining its impact on chronic diseases, inflammation, and the immune system. Understanding this aspect of the vagus nerve will help you leverage its full potential in the pursuit of overall health and wellness.

Chapter 4: The Healing Power of the Vagus Nerve

The vagus nerve, often referred to as the body's "superhighway," plays a vital role in maintaining health and well-being. Not only does it regulate many of our automatic bodily functions, but it also holds great potential for healing. In this chapter, we will explore the profound healing power of the vagus nerve, particularly in relation to chronic diseases, inflammation, and immune function. By understanding how the vagus nerve influences the body's recovery and defense mechanisms, we can harness its potential to promote healing, restore balance, and support overall health.

The Vagus Nerve as a Tool for Healing

The vagus nerve is an essential component of the parasympathetic nervous system, which governs the body's "rest and digest" functions. When activated, it calms the body, lowers stress levels, and fosters recovery. This healing effect occurs through several mechanisms that directly affect inflammation, heart rate, digestion, and immune function. One of the most significant ways the vagus nerve contributes to healing is through its ability to regulate the inflammatory response.

Inflammation is the body's natural defense mechanism against infection or injury. However, chronic inflammation is at the root of many modern health conditions, including autoimmune diseases, cardiovascular disease, and even depression. The vagus nerve helps prevent this chronic inflammation by sending signals to the brain that control the release of anti-inflammatory molecules.

By stimulating the vagus nerve, we can activate a natural anti-inflammatory response that mitigates the impact of long-term, low-grade inflammation in the body. This can be particularly beneficial in treating conditions like arthritis, inflammatory bowel disease (IBD), and other chronic inflammatory conditions.

In recent years, **vagus nerve stimulation (VNS)** has emerged as a therapeutic technique that uses electrical impulses to activate the vagus nerve. This technique has been shown to have promising results in reducing inflammation and improving outcomes in various medical conditions, including rheumatoid arthritis, Crohn's disease, and even certain neurological disorders. However, there are also non-invasive ways to stimulate the vagus nerve through lifestyle practices like deep breathing, meditation, and cold exposure, which can also help support the body's natural healing processes.

The Impact on Chronic Diseases and Inflammation

Chronic diseases, which are often driven by prolonged inflammation, are among the leading causes of death and disability worldwide. These diseases include conditions such as heart disease, diabetes, chronic respiratory diseases, and autoimmune conditions. One of the primary ways the vagus nerve helps combat chronic diseases is by modulating the inflammatory response.

When the vagus nerve is activated, it triggers the **cholinergic anti-inflammatory pathway**, a mechanism that reduces the production of pro-inflammatory cytokines and promotes the release of anti-inflammatory molecules. This process is crucial in preventing the escalation of chronic inflammation, which can damage tissues and lead to disease progression.

In studies involving **vagus nerve stimulation (VNS)**, patients with conditions like rheumatoid arthritis and Crohn's disease have reported significant reductions in inflammation and improved symptoms. For instance, VNS has been shown to decrease levels of inflammatory markers like TNF-alpha and IL-6, which are implicated in many chronic diseases.

Additionally, the vagus nerve's ability to influence the brain and gut provides a holistic approach to managing inflammation. The **gut-brain axis**, a communication pathway between the gut and the central nervous system, is influenced by the vagus nerve, and imbalances in this system have been linked to conditions like IBS, IBD, and even mental health disorders. By stimulating the vagus nerve, we can restore balance in the gut-brain axis, improve digestive health, and reduce inflammation, ultimately promoting healing from within.

The Vagus Nerve and Immunity: Strengthening Your Defenses

The immune system is the body's primary defense mechanism against infection and disease. The vagus nerve plays a critical role in regulating immune function, particularly through its ability to control inflammation and modulate immune responses. As mentioned earlier, the vagus nerve activates the cholinergic anti-inflammatory pathway, which helps prevent excessive inflammation that can damage tissues and lead to autoimmune diseases.

In addition to regulating inflammation, the vagus nerve also enhances the body's ability to fight infection. By stimulating the vagus nerve, we can improve the immune response, allowing the body to more effectively combat pathogens and prevent illness. This is particularly relevant in the context of viral infections, where the body's immune system can become overwhelmed by the inflammatory response.

Researchers are exploring the potential of vagus nerve stimulation as a treatment for immune-related diseases, such as rheumatoid arthritis, Crohn's disease, and even sepsis. By harnessing the vagus nerve's ability to modulate inflammation and immune responses, we may be able to develop new treatments for conditions that involve immune system dysfunction.

Healing Chronic Pain with the Vagus Nerve

Chronic pain is a debilitating condition that affects millions of people worldwide. Pain is often the result of inflammation or nerve damage, and it can significantly impact a person's quality of life. The vagus nerve has been shown to play a role in regulating pain perception and managing chronic pain.

One of the mechanisms through which the vagus nerve affects pain is through its influence on the **autonomic nervous system**, which controls involuntary functions like heart rate, blood pressure, and respiration. Chronic pain often involves an overactive sympathetic nervous system, which is responsible for the "fight or flight" response. By stimulating the vagus nerve, we can activate the parasympathetic nervous system, which counteracts the effects of the sympathetic system and promotes relaxation, pain relief, and healing.

Vagus nerve stimulation has been explored as a potential treatment for chronic pain conditions, including fibromyalgia, migraines, and neuropathic pain. Research has shown that stimulating the vagus nerve can help reduce pain intensity and improve overall pain management. Non-invasive techniques like deep breathing and meditation can also provide pain relief by activating the vagus nerve and encouraging the body's natural pain regulation mechanisms.

Practical Ways to Harness the Healing Power of the Vagus Nerve

While **vagus nerve stimulation (VNS)** therapy is an effective treatment for many conditions, there are several non-invasive methods that individuals can use to stimulate the vagus nerve and promote healing. These methods can be incorporated into daily life to improve overall health and well-being:

1. **Deep Breathing and Diaphragmatic Breathing**: Slow, deep breathing activates the vagus nerve and engages the parasympathetic nervous system, promoting relaxation and reducing inflammation. Focus on breathing deeply into your diaphragm rather than shallow chest breathing.
2. **Meditation and Mindfulness**: Meditation practices, especially those focused on breath control and body awareness, can help stimulate the vagus nerve. Mindfulness practices help activate the parasympathetic nervous system, reduce stress, and promote healing.
3. **Cold Exposure**: Cold therapy, such as taking cold showers or splashing your face with cold water, can activate the vagus nerve and trigger the body's relaxation response. Cold exposure has been shown to reduce inflammation and improve immune function.
4. **Yoga**: Yoga is a powerful practice that combines deep breathing, movement, and mindfulness. Certain poses, such as the shoulder stand and headstand, can help stimulate the vagus nerve and enhance parasympathetic activity.
5. **Social Connection and Positive Touch**: Engaging in positive social interactions, hugging, or even petting an animal can activate the vagus nerve. These social bonding activities promote emotional well-being and contribute to healing by enhancing vagal tone.

6. **Regular Exercise**: Physical activity, especially aerobic exercise, can improve vagal tone and help regulate inflammation. Exercise also promotes circulation, which supports overall immune function and healing.

Conclusion

The vagus nerve is an essential tool for healing. Through its powerful effects on inflammation, immune regulation, and pain management, the vagus nerve plays a central role in restoring balance and promoting recovery within the body. Whether through direct vagus nerve stimulation (VNS) or simple, everyday practices like deep breathing, yoga, and cold exposure, we can activate the vagus nerve to support healing from chronic diseases, reduce inflammation, and strengthen the immune system.

By mastering the vagus nerve and understanding its healing potential, we can take an active role in our own recovery and well-being. In the next chapter, we will explore the connection between the vagus nerve and mental health, examining how the vagus nerve influences emotional regulation and how we can use vagal techniques to restore balance in our emotional lives.

Chapter 5: The Vagus Nerve and Mental Health

Mental health disorders, including depression, anxiety, and post-traumatic stress disorder (PTSD), are among the most prevalent and debilitating health conditions in the world today. Many of these conditions are linked to dysregulation within the autonomic nervous system (ANS), particularly to a dysfunction of the parasympathetic nervous system, of which the vagus nerve is a key player. In this chapter, we will explore the role the vagus nerve plays in mental health, examine how vagal tone impacts emotional well-being, and discuss how stimulating the vagus nerve can be a transformative approach to restoring balance to the mind and body.

Depression, Anxiety, and PTSD: A Vagal Dysfunction Connection

Over the past few decades, research has revealed a fascinating connection between vagal dysfunction and various mental health conditions. The vagus nerve, as the primary nerve of the parasympathetic nervous system, plays a crucial role in the body's ability to regulate emotions and respond to stress. Low vagal tone, or a reduced ability of the vagus nerve to activate the parasympathetic nervous system, has been consistently linked to depression, anxiety, and PTSD.

Depression is often characterized by persistent feelings of sadness, hopelessness, and a lack of energy or motivation. Chronic inflammation, a common feature of depression, has been shown to decrease vagal tone. The vagus nerve helps to regulate inflammation by signaling the brain to release anti-inflammatory cytokines, so when vagal activity is low, this anti-inflammatory effect is impaired, contributing to the severity of depressive symptoms.

Anxiety disorders, including generalized anxiety and panic attacks, are also closely associated with low vagal tone. The vagus nerve helps to counterbalance the body's stress response, which is controlled by the sympathetic nervous system. When vagal activity is low, the body remains in a state of heightened arousal, making it difficult to regulate anxiety and stress levels. The inability to shift from the "fight or flight" mode to "rest and digest" contributes to feelings of unease and panic.

PTSD is another condition where vagal dysfunction plays a significant role. PTSD is typically triggered by traumatic events and is characterized by persistent fear, flashbacks, and hyperarousal. The body's inability to shift from a constant state of heightened alertness (sympathetic dominance) to a calm, restorative state (parasympathetic dominance) is thought to be related to vagus nerve dysfunction. A compromised vagal tone reduces the ability to calm the body's stress response, making it more difficult to heal emotionally from trauma.

How Vagal Tone Impacts Mental Well-Being

Vagal tone refers to the activity of the vagus nerve and its ability to regulate the autonomic nervous system, particularly in terms of the parasympathetic response. A higher vagal tone indicates that the parasympathetic nervous system is functioning efficiently, enabling the body to recover from stress, regulate emotions, and promote relaxation. On the other hand, low vagal tone is often associated with poor emotional regulation, increased stress levels, and a heightened vulnerability to mental health disorders.

The vagus nerve's ability to regulate the heart rate is one of the key indicators of vagal tone. Heart rate variability (HRV), the variation in time between heartbeats, is a direct measure of vagal tone. High HRV indicates good vagal function and a body that can efficiently shift between states of relaxation and arousal. Low HRV, on the other hand, is a sign of low vagal tone and is commonly seen in individuals with depression, anxiety, and PTSD. Low HRV has also been associated with increased risk of cardiovascular disease and other stress-related health conditions.

Researchers have found that improving vagal tone through various techniques can improve mental health outcomes. For example, increasing vagal activity has been shown to enhance emotional regulation, improve mood, and reduce symptoms of anxiety and depression. By stimulating the vagus nerve, we can restore the body's natural ability to manage stress and improve overall emotional well-being.

Restoring Balance: A Vagus Nerve Approach to Mental Health

The good news is that vagal tone is not static—it is modifiable. A variety of practices have been shown to effectively stimulate the vagus nerve, restore parasympathetic balance, and improve mental health. In this section, we will explore some of the most effective ways to activate the vagus nerve and enhance emotional well-being.

1. **Deep Breathing Exercises**:

   One of the simplest and most effective ways to activate the vagus nerve is through **deep breathing**. Slow, deep breaths—particularly diaphragmatic breathing, where the belly rises and falls with each inhale and exhale—help stimulate the vagus nerve and activate the parasympathetic nervous system. Breathing exercises can reduce heart rate, lower blood pressure, and promote a state of calm, all of which are beneficial for mental health. The **4-7-8 breathing technique**, where you inhale for 4 seconds, hold for 7 seconds, and exhale for 8 seconds, is particularly effective at increasing vagal tone.

2. **Mindfulness Meditation**:

   Meditation practices, particularly mindfulness and loving-kindness meditation, have been shown to activate the vagus nerve. These practices involve focusing on the present moment, observing thoughts without judgment, and cultivating feelings of compassion and gratitude. Research has shown that mindfulness meditation can increase vagal tone, improve mood, reduce stress, and enhance emotional regulation.

3. **Yoga**:

    Yoga is another powerful tool for stimulating the vagus nerve. The combination of controlled breathing, movement, and mindfulness in yoga promotes parasympathetic activation and enhances vagal tone. Certain yoga poses, such as **shoulder stand** or **child's pose**, can help stimulate the vagus nerve and foster a deeper sense of relaxation. Regular yoga practice has been shown to reduce symptoms of anxiety, depression, and PTSD.

4. **Cold Exposure**:

    Cold exposure is a more unconventional but highly effective method of stimulating the vagus nerve. Techniques like **cold showers** or splashing cold water on your face activate the body's parasympathetic response, lowering stress levels and improving vagal tone. Cold exposure has been shown to reduce inflammation and improve mood by triggering the vagus nerve to release anti-inflammatory compounds.

5. **Social Connection and Positive Touch**:

    Engaging in positive social interactions, whether through conversation, hugs, or simply spending time with loved ones, can stimulate the vagus nerve and promote emotional well-being. Research has shown that social support and physical touch are associated with increased vagal tone, making social connection a crucial part of maintaining mental health. Building strong relationships and having a support network can help reduce the impact of stress, anxiety, and depression.

6. **Vagus Nerve Stimulation (VNS) Therapy**:

   For individuals suffering from treatment-resistant depression or PTSD, **vagus nerve stimulation (VNS)** therapy is an FDA-approved medical treatment. VNS involves surgically implanting a device that sends electrical impulses to the vagus nerve, increasing vagal activity and promoting parasympathetic balance. Clinical studies have shown that VNS therapy can significantly reduce symptoms of depression and anxiety in patients who do not respond to traditional medications.

Practical Tips for Enhancing Mental Health with Vagal Stimulation

- **Create a Daily Breathing Practice**: Dedicate a few minutes each day to deep breathing exercises, such as diaphragmatic breathing or the 4-7-8 method. This simple practice can be done anywhere and can significantly improve vagal tone over time.
- **Engage in Regular Meditation**: Set aside time each day for meditation or mindfulness practice. Apps like Headspace or Calm offer guided meditation sessions that are designed to activate the vagus nerve and enhance emotional resilience.
- **Incorporate Yoga into Your Routine**: If you don't already practice yoga, consider starting with gentle poses that emphasize breathing and relaxation. Classes or online tutorials are great ways to get started and learn the fundamentals of yoga.
- **Embrace Cold Exposure**: Start by splashing cold water on your face or taking a quick cold shower. Gradually increase your tolerance to cold exposure over time. The shock to the body activates the vagus nerve, stimulating a sense of calm.
- **Strengthen Social Connections**: Make an effort to spend quality time with loved ones, whether through social activities or physical touch. Positive social interactions are key to mental well-being and support vagal activation.

Conclusion

The vagus nerve is a powerful tool in the regulation of mental health. From its ability to modulate stress and inflammation to its influence on emotional resilience and social bonding, the vagus nerve plays a vital role in maintaining mental well-being. By understanding how vagal tone affects mental health and implementing strategies to activate the vagus nerve, we can effectively manage symptoms of depression, anxiety, PTSD, and other mental health conditions.

In the next chapter, we will explore how the vagus nerve can be used as a tool for physical healing, particularly in relation to chronic diseases and inflammation. Through a deeper understanding of the vagus nerve's healing potential, we will continue to unlock new ways to optimize our health and well-being.

Chapter 6: Breathing Techniques to Stimulate the Vagus Nerve

The breath is not only vital for life—it also serves as a powerful tool for influencing the body's autonomic nervous system (ANS), particularly the parasympathetic nervous system, in which the vagus nerve plays a central role. Through the breath, we can activate the vagus nerve, promoting relaxation, reducing stress, and enhancing overall health. In this chapter, we will explore the science behind breathing techniques that stimulate the vagus nerve, and how incorporating these practices into daily life can improve both physical and mental well-being.

The Role of Breathing in Vagus Nerve Activation

The vagus nerve is often referred to as the "rest and digest" nerve, and it is responsible for slowing the heart rate, lowering blood pressure, and promoting relaxation. It is the primary nerve that helps the body recover from stress and maintain homeostasis. When the vagus nerve is activated, it triggers the parasympathetic nervous system, which calms the body and counters the effects of the sympathetic nervous system, the system responsible for the "fight or flight" stress response.

Breathing is a simple yet effective way to stimulate the vagus nerve. Slow, deep breathing engages the diaphragm, which activates the vagus nerve and enhances vagal tone. The vagus nerve responds to the rhythm and depth of your breath, and by consciously slowing and deepening your breathing, you signal to your body that it is time to relax, thereby reducing the physiological markers of stress.

Several studies have shown that slow, controlled breathing increases heart rate variability (HRV), which is a direct indicator of vagal tone. Higher HRV is associated with better emotional regulation, greater resilience to stress, and overall improved health. By using specific breathing techniques, we can enhance vagal activity and improve our ability to manage stress and emotional fluctuations.

Deep Breathing Exercises

One of the most effective ways to activate the vagus nerve is through **deep breathing**. Deep breathing focuses on filling the lungs fully, using the diaphragm rather than shallow chest breathing. When the diaphragm moves downward during inhalation, it increases vagal tone, leading to relaxation.

The 4-7-8 Breathing Technique

One of the most well-known deep breathing techniques that can stimulate the vagus nerve is the **4-7-8 technique**. This method involves controlling the breath in a specific pattern to promote relaxation and enhance vagal activation:

1. **Inhale** through your nose for 4 seconds, filling your lungs deeply from your diaphragm.
2. **Hold** the breath for 7 seconds.
3. **Exhale** slowly through your mouth for 8 seconds, letting all the air out and relaxing your body with each exhalation.

This technique works by slowing down the breath, which in turn calms the nervous system. The key to this exercise is making the exhalation longer than the inhalation, which naturally activates the parasympathetic system. Practicing this technique for just a few minutes each day can help reduce anxiety, improve sleep quality, and enhance overall vagal tone.

Box Breathing (Square Breathing)

Another powerful technique for vagal stimulation is **box breathing** or **square breathing**, which involves holding each phase of the breath for equal intervals. This technique is widely used by athletes and high-stress professionals to improve focus and calm the nervous system. Here's how you do it:

1. **Inhale** through your nose for 4 seconds.
2. **Hold** the breath for 4 seconds.
3. **Exhale** slowly through your mouth for 4 seconds.
4. **Hold** the breath again for 4 seconds before repeating the cycle.

Box breathing helps to regulate the breath, slowing it down and increasing vagal tone by ensuring that each phase of the breathing cycle is equally long. This practice can help reduce feelings of stress and tension, promote mental clarity, and create a sense of balance and control.

Diaphragmatic Breathing: Activating the Vagus Nerve

Diaphragmatic breathing, also known as **abdominal breathing**, is another effective way to activate the vagus nerve and promote relaxation. Unlike chest breathing, which only fills the upper part of the lungs, diaphragmatic breathing focuses on engaging the diaphragm to fill the lungs fully. This type of breathing is particularly powerful because it activates the parasympathetic nervous system, helping to calm the body and improve emotional regulation.

To practice diaphragmatic breathing:

1. **Sit comfortably** with your back straight or lie down on your back.
2. **Place one hand on your chest** and the other on your abdomen.
3. **Take a slow, deep breath in** through your nose, allowing your abdomen to rise as the diaphragm moves downward.
4. **Exhale slowly** through your mouth, feeling your abdomen fall with each exhale. Try to keep your chest as still as possible during the process.
5. Continue this pattern for several minutes, focusing on the rise and fall of your abdomen.

Diaphragmatic breathing can be done anywhere and anytime, and it can help reduce anxiety, promote deeper sleep, and improve overall vagal tone. For optimal results, aim to practice diaphragmatic breathing for 5–10 minutes daily.

Breathing for Relaxation and Stress Relief

When it comes to using breathing to manage stress, the focus should be on slowing down the breath and deepening each inhale and exhale. Here are a few additional techniques for stress relief:

Resonant or Coherent Breathing

- Inhale for 5 seconds.
- Exhale for 5 seconds.
- Repeat for several minutes, aiming for a smooth and even rhythm.

Alternate Nostril Breathing (Nadi Shodhana)

- Sit in a comfortable position and close your eyes.
- Use your right thumb to close off your right nostril.
- Inhale deeply and slowly through your left nostril.
- Close your left nostril with your right ring finger and release your right nostril.
- Exhale slowly through your right nostril.
- Inhale through your right nostril, then close it and exhale through your left nostril.
- Repeat for several minutes.

Alternate nostril breathing has been shown to improve vagal tone, reduce stress, and enhance overall well-being by promoting balance in the autonomic nervous system.

Practical Tips for Incorporating Breathing Techniques

1. **Start Small**: If you're new to these techniques, begin with just a few minutes of breathing practice each day. Over time, you can gradually increase the duration to 10–20 minutes per session.
2. **Be Consistent**: Like any other habit, breathing exercises are most effective when practiced regularly. Set aside time each day for your breathing practice, ideally in the morning or before bed, to improve overall vagal tone.
3. **Use Breathing as a Stress Management Tool**: Whenever you feel stressed, anxious, or overwhelmed, take a moment to practice one of the breathing techniques outlined in this chapter. Even a minute of deep, slow breathing can help shift your body out of a stress response and into a more relaxed, balanced state.
4. **Combine with Other Practices**: Breathing techniques can be paired with other vagus nerve-stimulating practices such as meditation, yoga, or mindfulness. This combination amplifies the benefits for stress relief and emotional regulation.

Conclusion

Breathing is one of the most accessible and effective tools we have for activating the vagus nerve and promoting relaxation. By mastering deep breathing, diaphragmatic breathing, and other focused breathing techniques, we can stimulate the vagus nerve, reduce stress, and enhance emotional and physical well-being. These practices are simple to incorporate into daily life and offer profound benefits for mental health, stress management, and overall health.

In the next chapter, we will explore how meditation and mindfulness can further enhance vagus nerve function, improve emotional regulation, and contribute to a more balanced and resilient nervous system.

Chapter 7: Meditation and Mindfulness: Rewiring the Vagus Nerve

Meditation and mindfulness practices have long been recognized for their ability to calm the mind, reduce stress, and enhance emotional regulation. More recently, research has uncovered the profound effects these practices can have on the vagus nerve, the body's primary mechanism for relaxation and stress recovery. By consciously engaging in meditation and mindfulness, we can activate the vagus nerve, improve vagal tone, and promote a state of balance in both body and mind. In this chapter, we will explore how meditation and mindfulness help "rewire" the vagus nerve and why these practices are indispensable for achieving optimal health and emotional well-being.

The Role of Meditation in Vagus Nerve Health

Meditation is a mental discipline that focuses the mind and encourages the individual to remain in a state of heightened awareness or presence. The core purpose of meditation is to achieve mental clarity, emotional balance, and relaxation. It turns out that these mental states are not just good for the mind but also have profound physical effects, particularly on the vagus nerve.

Through regular meditation practice, we can strengthen the parasympathetic nervous system, where the vagus nerve is the principal player. When activated, the vagus nerve promotes relaxation, slowing the heart rate, reducing blood pressure, and encouraging the body's recovery from stress. By inducing a state of calm through meditation, we trigger vagus nerve activation, which, in turn, can enhance vagal tone.

Studies have shown that meditation increases heart rate variability (HRV), a direct measure of vagal tone. High HRV indicates a strong, responsive parasympathetic system, which is associated with greater emotional resilience, better stress management, and improved overall health. Meditation is one of the most effective and accessible ways to activate the vagus nerve and increase HRV, thereby improving both physical and mental health.

The Science Behind Meditation and Vagal Tone

The connection between meditation and vagal tone lies in the ability of meditation to slow down physiological processes, such as the heart rate and breath rate, both of which are governed by the autonomic nervous system (ANS). The vagus nerve plays a key role in controlling these functions, and when we meditate, we activate the parasympathetic nervous system, which is responsible for relaxation.

During meditation, particularly deep-breathing meditations, the vagus nerve is stimulated, leading to a reduction in the "fight or flight" response driven by the sympathetic nervous system. This shift allows the body to enter a state of calm, making it easier for the mind to focus and for emotions to stabilize.

A significant amount of research has shown that practices like mindfulness meditation, guided breathing, and loving-kindness meditation can increase vagal tone by stimulating the vagus nerve. These meditative techniques focus on breath, awareness, and the present moment—all of which directly influence vagal activity and help restore balance to the nervous system.

Mindfulness Practices for Calming the Nervous System

Mindfulness is the practice of bringing one's attention to the present moment, without judgment. It involves observing thoughts, feelings, and bodily sensations with a sense of curiosity and acceptance, rather than reacting impulsively or trying to control them. Mindfulness practices are not only beneficial for mental health, but they also support the activation of the vagus nerve and the parasympathetic nervous system.

Mindfulness-based practices can take many forms, including body scans, mindful breathing, and mindful eating. These practices have been shown to enhance emotional regulation, improve focus, and reduce symptoms of anxiety and depression by boosting vagal tone.

Mindful Breathing: One of the simplest ways to activate the vagus nerve through mindfulness is to focus on the breath. The act of taking deep, slow breaths while maintaining awareness of the inhales and exhales signals the body to switch from the sympathetic stress response to the parasympathetic relaxation response. This practice helps to increase HRV and reduce stress hormones, promoting a sense of calm.

Body Scan Meditation: This form of mindfulness involves mentally scanning the body, starting from the tips of the toes and slowly moving up to the head. It encourages relaxation and awareness of physical sensations, helping to release tension stored in the body and activating the vagus nerve. By focusing on the body's sensations, the individual becomes more attuned to the signals of stress and learns how to relax more deeply.

Loving-Kindness Meditation (Metta): In loving-kindness meditation, practitioners focus on generating feelings of love, compassion, and goodwill, first for themselves and then for others. This type of meditation enhances the vagus nerve's ability to regulate emotional responses and has been shown to improve heart rate variability, reduce stress, and promote social connectedness.

Creating a Daily Meditation Practice for Long-Term Benefits

The benefits of meditation are cumulative—regular practice leads to lasting improvements in vagal tone, emotional resilience, and overall well-being. Here are some practical tips for creating a meditation routine that supports vagus nerve health:

1. **Start Small**: If you're new to meditation, begin with just a few minutes a day. As little as 5-10 minutes of mindful breathing or guided meditation can be enough to stimulate the vagus nerve and reduce stress.
2. **Set a Consistent Time**: Meditation is most effective when practiced consistently. Try to incorporate meditation into your daily routine, whether it's in the morning, during lunch breaks, or before bed. The key is to make it a habit.
3. **Focus on the Breath**: One of the simplest forms of meditation involves focusing solely on the breath. Breathe deeply and slowly, allowing the breath to move naturally through the body. Use counting or guided meditation apps to help maintain focus and enhance the practice.
4. **Use Guided Meditation**: If you find it challenging to meditate on your own, use guided meditation apps or audio recordings to help structure the practice. Many apps offer mindfulness sessions specifically designed to activate the vagus nerve and promote emotional balance.
5. **Practice Mindfulness in Everyday Activities**: Meditation doesn't have to be limited to a formal session. You can practice mindfulness throughout your day by paying full attention to whatever you're doing—whether it's eating, walking, or even washing the dishes. The more you practice mindfulness, the easier it will be to regulate your emotional state and engage your parasympathetic nervous system when needed.

6. **Be Patient**: The benefits of meditation take time to manifest. Be patient with yourself and recognize that each practice session, no matter how short, is contributing to improving your vagal tone and overall emotional health.

Long-Term Benefits of Meditation for the Vagus Nerve

As you develop a regular meditation practice, you may begin to notice significant changes in your overall well-being. These include:

- **Improved Emotional Regulation**: Meditation can help you respond more calmly to stressful situations and improve your ability to manage negative emotions like anxiety, anger, and sadness.

- **Reduced Symptoms of Anxiety and Depression**: Increased vagal tone resulting from meditation has been linked to reduced symptoms of anxiety and depression, making it an effective tool for improving mental health.

- **Enhanced Focus and Clarity**: Meditation helps improve cognitive function by enhancing focus, memory, and the ability to think clearly. These cognitive benefits are related to the calming effects of vagus nerve activation.

- **Better Sleep**: Meditation, particularly relaxation techniques before bedtime, can significantly improve sleep quality by calming the nervous system and preparing the body for restorative rest.

- **Stronger Immune Function**: Through its effects on the autonomic nervous system, meditation can enhance immune function by reducing inflammation and boosting the body's natural defenses.

Conclusion

Meditation and mindfulness practices offer a powerful way to activate the vagus nerve and enhance overall health. By slowing down the breath, calming the nervous system, and cultivating a deep sense of awareness, these practices promote relaxation, emotional regulation, and resilience to stress. Regular meditation and mindfulness practices can be transformative tools for improving vagal tone, reducing anxiety and depression, and enhancing both physical and mental well-being.

In the next chapter, we will explore the benefits of cold exposure for stimulating the vagus nerve, another effective way to improve health and well-being through the activation of the parasympathetic nervous system.

Chapter 8: Cold Exposure and the Vagus Nerve

When we think about ways to enhance health, cold exposure may not immediately come to mind. However, recent research has revealed the powerful impact that cold therapy can have on activating the vagus nerve and improving overall well-being. Cold exposure is a highly effective technique for stimulating the parasympathetic nervous system, where the vagus nerve plays a key role. In this chapter, we will explore how cold exposure stimulates the vagus nerve, the science behind it, and practical tips for incorporating cold therapy into your routine to maximize its health benefits.

How Cold Therapy Stimulates the Vagus Nerve

Cold exposure, whether through cold showers, ice baths, or even brief exposure to cold air, triggers a physiological response in the body known as the **cold shock response**. When the body is exposed to cold, it goes through several adaptive changes, one of which is the activation of the vagus nerve. The vagus nerve helps the body adapt to stress by promoting relaxation and restoring balance to the autonomic nervous system.

When exposed to cold temperatures, the body's **sympathetic nervous system** (the "fight or flight" response) initially kicks in. This is followed by a **parasympathetic rebound**, which is where the vagus nerve plays a key role. The vagus nerve activates the body's "rest and digest" functions, slowing down the heart rate, reducing inflammation, and promoting recovery.

Cold exposure also triggers the release of various hormones, such as norepinephrine and endorphins, which help improve mood, reduce pain, and promote healing. These biochemical responses, combined with the vagal stimulation, contribute to the many benefits of cold therapy.

The Science Behind Cold Showers and Ice Baths

The science behind cold exposure and its effects on the vagus nerve is rooted in its ability to stimulate the **autonomic nervous system (ANS)**, which controls involuntary bodily functions. The ANS has two primary branches: the sympathetic nervous system (responsible for the "fight or flight" response) and the parasympathetic nervous system (responsible for the "rest and digest" functions).

Cold exposure activates the sympathetic system initially, but after this acute stress response, the parasympathetic system is activated, and this is where the vagus nerve comes into play. Specifically, cold exposure helps to increase **heart rate variability (HRV)**, a measure of the time variation between heartbeats. High HRV is associated with better vagal tone and overall resilience to stress. By stimulating the vagus nerve, cold exposure helps to balance the autonomic nervous system, making the body more adaptable to stress and promoting relaxation.

One study published in *Psychosomatic Medicine* found that cold exposure, particularly through methods like ice baths, led to an increase in **vagal tone** and a reduction in **sympathetic nervous system activity**. This means that not only does cold exposure activate the vagus nerve, but it also enhances the body's ability to recover from stress and return to a calm state more quickly.

Practical Tips for Incorporating Cold Exposure

Cold exposure doesn't have to mean plunging into an ice bath (although that's an option if you're brave!). There are a variety of ways to incorporate cold therapy into your routine that are both effective and accessible.

1. **Cold Showers**: One of the simplest and most accessible methods for cold exposure is taking a cold shower. Start by gradually reducing the temperature of your shower to a colder setting at the end of your usual shower. Begin with 30 seconds to a minute of cold water exposure, and gradually increase the time as your body adapts. The cold shower activates the vagus nerve, which helps the body shift into a relaxed state.

2. **Ice Baths**: If you're more accustomed to cold exposure, ice baths are another powerful way to activate the vagus nerve. To take an ice bath, fill a bathtub with cold water and add ice. Start with just a few minutes of immersion and gradually build up to 10–15 minutes. While this can be intense, the benefits are profound, especially in terms of reducing muscle soreness, improving recovery, and enhancing vagal tone.

3. **Cold Face Immersion**: A less intense but still effective method of cold exposure is to immerse your face in cold water. Simply fill a bowl with cold water and ice, and submerge your face for 20–30 seconds. This technique, known as the **diving reflex**, stimulates the vagus nerve and helps to reduce heart rate, improve circulation, and promote relaxation.

4. **Cold Exposure in Nature**: If you live in a cold climate, you can also expose your body to cold air by spending time outdoors in cold weather. A brisk walk in the cold can activate the vagus nerve and boost overall health. Be sure to dress appropriately for the weather to avoid hypothermia.

5. **Cryotherapy**: For those who have access to cryotherapy centers, this method involves exposing the body to extremely cold air for a short period (usually 2-3 minutes) in a controlled environment. Cryotherapy has been shown to reduce inflammation, enhance recovery, and activate the vagus nerve.

How Cold Exposure Benefits the Vagus Nerve

In addition to activating the vagus nerve, cold exposure has numerous benefits for overall health and well-being:

1. **Reduces Inflammation**: Cold exposure stimulates the vagus nerve's ability to regulate inflammation. By activating the parasympathetic nervous system, it can help reduce inflammation in the body, making it an effective strategy for managing chronic pain, arthritis, and other inflammatory conditions.
2. **Improves Mood**: Cold exposure triggers the release of endorphins, the body's natural "feel-good" hormones. These neurochemicals help elevate mood and reduce feelings of depression or anxiety. Regular cold exposure has been linked to improved mood and mental clarity, especially in individuals with mood disorders.
3. **Boosts Immune Function**: Cold exposure strengthens the immune system by increasing white blood cell count and promoting circulation. As the vagus nerve is activated, it also helps to reduce inflammation and regulate immune responses, making the body more efficient at fighting infections and healing.
4. **Improves Cardiovascular Health**: Cold exposure helps to enhance heart rate variability (HRV), an indicator of vagal tone and cardiovascular health. Higher HRV is associated with better heart health, increased resilience to stress, and improved emotional regulation.
5. **Promotes Recovery**: Athletes and fitness enthusiasts often use ice baths and cold showers to speed up recovery after intense physical activity. Cold exposure reduces muscle inflammation, enhances circulation, and accelerates the removal of waste products like lactic acid from the muscles.

6. **Increases Alertness**: Cold exposure can also boost energy and alertness. The shock from cold water increases the production of norepinephrine, a neurotransmitter that helps improve focus, attention, and overall cognitive function.

How to Integrate Cold Exposure into Daily Life

To start benefiting from cold exposure, begin gradually and listen to your body. Here are a few tips for safely incorporating cold therapy into your routine:

- **Start Slow**: If you're new to cold exposure, start with shorter durations and lower temperatures. Begin with cold showers and gradually increase the duration or intensity as your body becomes accustomed to the cold.
- **Use a Systematic Approach**: Practice cold exposure in a structured manner, such as alternating between 30 seconds of cold exposure followed by a few minutes of normal temperature or warm water. This will help your body adapt to the cold in a manageable way.
- **Be Consistent**: To see the best results, incorporate cold exposure into your daily routine. Even small amounts of exposure can make a big difference in terms of activating the vagus nerve and improving overall health.
- **Monitor Your Body's Response**: Pay attention to how your body responds to cold exposure. If you feel lightheaded or experience pain, stop immediately and warm up. Cold exposure should feel invigorating, not painful.

Conclusion

Cold exposure is a powerful and accessible way to activate the vagus nerve and unlock its full potential. Whether through cold showers, ice baths, or even cold face immersion, regularly incorporating cold therapy into your routine can improve emotional regulation, enhance recovery, boost immune function, and promote overall well-being. The vagus nerve plays a critical role in managing stress and inflammation, and cold exposure helps optimize its function for better health.

In the next chapter, we will explore how physical exercise can also stimulate the vagus nerve, enhance vagal tone, and improve both physical and mental health. By combining cold exposure with other vagus nerve-stimulating practices, we can create a comprehensive approach to health and vitality.

Chapter 9: Physical Exercise and Vagus Nerve Activation

Physical exercise is widely known for its benefits to overall health: it helps to control weight, strengthen the heart, and improve mental well-being. But did you know that regular physical activity can also enhance the function of your vagus nerve? As one of the central elements of the parasympathetic nervous system, the vagus nerve plays a critical role in regulating stress, controlling heart rate, and supporting the body's recovery processes. In this chapter, we will explore how physical exercise activates the vagus nerve, boosts vagal tone, and provides both immediate and long-term benefits for your health.

The Importance of Physical Movement for Vagal Tone

Vagal tone refers to the activity of the vagus nerve and its ability to regulate the autonomic nervous system (ANS). A strong vagal tone indicates that the parasympathetic nervous system (the "rest and digest" system) is effectively counterbalancing the stress responses initiated by the sympathetic nervous system (the "fight or flight" system). High vagal tone is associated with better emotional regulation, improved cardiovascular health, and greater resilience to stress.

Physical exercise is one of the most effective ways to enhance vagal tone. When we engage in physical activity, especially aerobic exercises, it triggers multiple physiological responses that stimulate the vagus nerve and improve its function. These responses include:

1. **Increased Heart Rate Variability (HRV)**: HRV is a key marker of vagal tone and overall heart health. During exercise, heart rate variability typically increases, signaling the activation of the vagus nerve. Regular exercise has been shown to boost HRV over time, leading to improved autonomic regulation and better cardiovascular health.
2. **Enhanced Parasympathetic Activity**: Exercise causes the body to shift from a state of rest to an active state, which initially activates the sympathetic nervous system. However, post-exercise, the vagus nerve kicks in, helping the body return to a restful state, reducing heart rate and promoting recovery. Regular exercise helps improve the efficiency of this transition and encourages a quicker recovery post-activity.
3. **Improved Stress Resilience**: Physical exercise helps to increase the body's tolerance to stress by enhancing vagal function. The more consistently you exercise, the better your body can handle stress, recover from physical exertion, and regulate emotional responses.

Activities That Boost Vagus Nerve Health

Not all exercises are equally effective for vagal tone. While any form of physical activity can contribute to overall health, certain types of exercise have been shown to be especially beneficial for stimulating the vagus nerve and improving vagal tone. Here are some of the best activities for vagus nerve activation:

Aerobic Exercise

running, swimming, cycling, and brisk walking

How to incorporate aerobic exercise

Yoga

How to incorporate yoga

Strength Training

strength training

How to incorporate strength training

Tai Chi and Qigong

How to incorporate Tai Chi or Qigong

Exercise Routines That Enhance Vagal Function

Creating a well-rounded exercise routine that incorporates a mix of aerobic exercise, strength training, and mindfulness practices like yoga or Tai Chi can provide the maximum benefits for vagal tone. Here's an example of a weekly routine that balances different types of exercise for optimal vagus nerve activation:

1. **Monday**: 30 minutes of brisk walking or light jogging (aerobic exercise) + 20 minutes of strength training (bodyweight exercises or weights)
2. **Tuesday**: 45 minutes of yoga or Tai Chi (mindfulness and vagal activation)
3. **Wednesday**: 30 minutes of cycling or swimming (aerobic exercise)
4. **Thursday**: Rest day or light stretching and deep breathing exercises
5. **Friday**: 30 minutes of running or cycling (aerobic exercise) + 20 minutes of strength training (resistance bands or weights)
6. **Saturday**: 45 minutes of yoga or Tai Chi + a short walk (mindfulness and relaxation)
7. **Sunday**: Rest day with optional light stretching or relaxation exercises

This balanced approach allows you to stimulate the vagus nerve through various forms of exercise, improving vagal tone, reducing stress, and promoting overall health.

The Connection Between Exercise and Emotional Well-Being

The benefits of physical exercise extend beyond just physical health—regular movement also plays a significant role in improving mental health. Exercise has been shown to reduce symptoms of depression and anxiety, partly due to its effects on the vagus nerve. By enhancing vagal tone, exercise helps the body recover from stress and return to a calm, balanced state.

Moreover, exercise stimulates the release of endorphins, the body's natural mood-boosting chemicals, contributing to better emotional regulation and a sense of well-being. This is why exercise is often considered a natural antidepressant, improving mood, reducing anxiety, and enhancing resilience to stress.

How to Integrate Exercise into Your Daily Life

To get the most out of physical activity for vagus nerve stimulation, consistency is key. Here are some tips for integrating exercise into your daily routine:

1. **Find Activities You Enjoy**: The best way to stick with exercise is to choose activities that you enjoy. Whether it's dancing, swimming, hiking, or playing a sport, find what excites you and incorporate it into your schedule.
2. **Start Small and Build Up**: If you're new to regular exercise, start with shorter sessions and gradually increase the intensity and duration. Even 10-15 minutes of moderate activity can have a positive impact on vagal tone.
3. **Set Realistic Goals**: Set achievable goals that motivate you. Whether it's walking for 30 minutes a day or completing a full yoga session, small milestones will help keep you on track and improve your consistency.
4. **Combine Exercise with Mindfulness**: Try pairing physical activity with mindfulness practices like deep breathing or meditation. This combination enhances both physical and emotional well-being, providing a holistic approach to vagal tone activation.

Conclusion

Physical exercise is one of the most effective and accessible ways to stimulate the vagus nerve and improve vagal tone. By incorporating aerobic exercise, strength training, yoga, and mindfulness practices into your routine, you can enhance emotional resilience, reduce stress, and improve overall health. Exercise not only strengthens the body but also supports the nervous system, enabling you to better manage stress, maintain emotional balance, and foster a greater sense of well-being.

In the next chapter, we will explore how nutrition plays a vital role in supporting vagus nerve function and overall health, emphasizing the connection between gut health, the vagus nerve, and your overall vitality.

Chapter 10: Nutrition and the Vagus Nerve

The vagus nerve is a critical player in regulating many bodily functions, including digestion, heart rate, and inflammation. As a key component of the parasympathetic nervous system, its primary role is to promote relaxation and recovery after stress. What many don't realize, however, is that the food we eat has a significant impact on vagal tone, and in turn, on our overall health. In this chapter, we will explore the connection between nutrition and vagus nerve health, how gut health influences the vagus nerve, and the best foods to support vagal tone and enhance well-being.

Foods That Support Vagus Nerve Health

Certain nutrients and foods have been shown to promote healthy vagal function by supporting the autonomic nervous system, reducing inflammation, and improving gut health—key factors that affect vagal tone. While no single food directly "stimulates" the vagus nerve, a balanced diet rich in anti-inflammatory, gut-healthy, and neuroprotective foods can enhance its activity and strengthen parasympathetic responses.

Here are some key nutrients and food categories that support vagus nerve health:

Omega-3 Fatty Acids

Sources

Probiotic-Rich Foods

Lactobacillus

Bifidobacterium

Sources

Polyphenols

Sources

Magnesium

Sources

Vitamin B12 and Folate

Sources

Amino Acids (L-Theanine and Tryptophan)

L-theanine

tryptophan

- **Sources of L-theanine**: Green tea, matcha, and some mushrooms.
- **Sources of tryptophan**: Turkey, chicken, eggs, nuts, seeds, and tofu.

Gut Health and the Vagus Nerve: The Connection

The gut-brain axis is the bidirectional communication network between the gut and the brain, and it is heavily influenced by the vagus nerve. About 90% of the signals from the gut to the brain are transmitted via the vagus nerve, and the state of the gut microbiome has a profound impact on vagal function.

Research has shown that a healthy, diverse gut microbiota not only supports proper digestion but also promotes a positive emotional state, enhances stress resilience, and improves immune function. Conversely, an imbalance in gut bacteria, known as **dysbiosis**, has been linked to a variety of health issues, including depression, anxiety, and inflammation—all of which can impair vagal function.

Supporting gut health through diet is essential for maintaining a healthy vagus nerve. Probiotic-rich foods (as mentioned above) and **prebiotics**—which feed beneficial gut bacteria—are crucial in fostering a healthy gut microbiome. Prebiotics are found in high-fiber foods that feed the good bacteria, promoting a balanced gut environment.

Sources of prebiotics

Additionally, **anti-inflammatory foods** such as turmeric, ginger, and omega-3-rich foods, can help combat the gut inflammation that often accompanies dysbiosis. Reducing chronic inflammation is key to supporting healthy vagus nerve activity and improving the gut-brain communication pathways.

How to Use Nutrition for Vagal Balance

1. **Eat a Whole-Food, Plant-Based Diet**: Focus on eating a variety of whole foods, especially vegetables, fruits, legumes, nuts, seeds, and whole grains. These foods are rich in fiber, antioxidants, vitamins, and minerals that support both gut health and nervous system function.
2. **Incorporate Healthy Fats**: Ensure that your diet includes healthy fats, especially omega-3 fatty acids, found in fatty fish and plant-based sources like flaxseeds and walnuts. These fats help reduce inflammation and support the brain and nervous system.
3. **Limit Processed Foods**: Highly processed foods, particularly those high in sugar and trans fats, can disrupt the gut microbiome, increase inflammation, and impair vagal function. Opt for whole, unprocessed foods whenever possible.
4. **Support Gut Health with Fermented Foods**: Include a variety of fermented foods in your diet to promote a healthy gut microbiome. These foods provide beneficial bacteria that help regulate digestion, reduce inflammation, and enhance vagus nerve function.
5. **Stay Hydrated**: Adequate hydration is essential for maintaining proper cellular function and promoting digestion. Drink plenty of water throughout the day to support the body's systems, including the vagus nerve's ability to regulate gut function.

6. **Avoid Gut Irritants**: Certain foods, such as processed sugars, alcohol, and artificial sweeteners, can disrupt gut health and contribute to inflammation. Reducing or eliminating these foods from your diet can help maintain a healthy gut-brain connection and improve vagal function.

Meal Plan for Vagus Nerve Support

To help you get started, here is an example of a day's meal plan designed to enhance vagus nerve function:

- **Breakfast**: A smoothie made with spinach, flaxseeds, berries, almond butter, and a scoop of protein powder (rich in tryptophan).
- **Lunch**: A salad with mixed greens, chickpeas, avocado, walnuts, olive oil, and lemon dressing (high in omega-3s and prebiotics).
- **Snack**: Greek yogurt (for probiotics) with a drizzle of honey and a sprinkle of chia seeds.
- **Dinner**: Grilled salmon (rich in omega-3s), quinoa, and steamed broccoli (packed with polyphenols and prebiotics).
- **Evening**: A cup of green tea (rich in L-theanine) before bed.

Conclusion

Nutrition plays a pivotal role in supporting the vagus nerve and enhancing its function. A diet rich in anti-inflammatory foods, probiotics, healthy fats, and gut-friendly nutrients can help improve vagal tone, strengthen the gut-brain connection, and promote overall well-being. By making mindful dietary choices, you can boost your vagus nerve health, reduce stress, and enhance resilience to emotional challenges.

In the next chapter, we will explore how music and sound can also activate the vagus nerve, offering yet another avenue for improving health and emotional balance through simple, enjoyable practices.

Chapter 11: Music, Sound, and the Vagus Nerve

Music and sound have been used for centuries across cultures for their therapeutic benefits. From ancient chants to modern sound therapies, sound has been a tool for promoting health, relaxation, and emotional well-being. Recent research has shown that certain sounds, frequencies, and even the act of singing or chanting can stimulate the vagus nerve, activating the parasympathetic nervous system and improving vagal tone. In this chapter, we will explore how music and sound can influence the vagus nerve, and how you can use sound as a powerful tool for enhancing your health and emotional regulation.

The Therapeutic Power of Music

Music has a profound impact on the human brain and body. From calming lullabies to powerful orchestral symphonies, music has the ability to alter mood, reduce stress, and influence physiological functions like heart rate, blood pressure, and respiration. These changes are not just psychological—music has tangible, measurable effects on the autonomic nervous system (ANS), which is controlled by the vagus nerve.

Music therapy has been shown to reduce stress, lower cortisol levels (the body's primary stress hormone), and increase parasympathetic activity (the "rest and digest" response), which is mediated by the vagus nerve. This explains why music is often used in therapeutic settings to help individuals cope with anxiety, depression, and chronic pain. When we listen to music, especially music that we enjoy, our body responds with relaxation and a reduction in stress levels, thanks to the vagus nerve's involvement in regulating the body's stress response.

One study published in *Frontiers in Psychology* found that listening to relaxing music increases HRV, a key marker of vagal tone, signaling that the vagus nerve is being activated. The positive effects of music on HRV are particularly notable in people experiencing high levels of stress, showing that music can be a powerful tool for emotional and physical recovery.

Using Sound to Stimulate the Vagus Nerve

In addition to music, other types of sound have been found to stimulate the vagus nerve. Sound frequencies, vibrations, and even the human voice have been shown to influence the autonomic nervous system and improve vagal tone.

Binaural Beats

How to incorporate binaural beats

Tuning Fork Therapy

How to incorporate tuning forks

Chanting and Singing

How to incorporate chanting and singing

The Role of Vibrational Sound Therapy

Beyond music and vocalization, vibrational sound therapies such as sound baths, gongs, and crystal bowls have gained popularity for their ability to promote relaxation and enhance vagal tone. These therapies work by creating vibrations that reverberate throughout the body, affecting both the mind and nervous system.

1. **Gong Baths**:

   Gong therapy uses the sound of large gongs to produce vibrations that resonate throughout the body. These vibrations have been shown to help reduce stress, improve sleep, and enhance vagus nerve activity. Gong baths have become a popular form of therapy in wellness centers around the world, where participants lie down and listen to the sound waves of the gong wash over them, creating deep states of relaxation and balance.

2. **Crystal Sound Bowls**:

   Crystal singing bowls produce pure, resonant tones that are believed to harmonize the body's energy fields. Many people find that these tones help reduce stress and improve mental clarity. Crystal bowls are often used in meditation settings to activate specific chakras, but they can also promote vagal activation and improve emotional well-being.

How to incorporate vibrational sound therapy

How to Incorporate Music and Sound into Your Routine

Incorporating music and sound therapy into your daily routine can be a simple and effective way to enhance vagal tone and improve emotional and physical health. Here are some practical ways to do so:

1. **Create a Calming Playlist**: Compile a playlist of relaxing music, nature sounds, or binaural beats to play during meditation, yoga, or before bed. Choose music that promotes relaxation and resonates with you personally. Classical, ambient, or instrumental music often works well for calming the nervous system.

2. **Sing or Hum Daily**: Start your day with a few minutes of humming or singing. This simple practice can help activate the vagus nerve, promote relaxation, and set a positive tone for the rest of the day.

3. **Attend Sound Therapy Sessions**: If you have access to sound therapists or wellness centers that offer gong baths, crystal bowl sound therapy, or vibrational sound sessions, consider attending regularly. These practices are deeply relaxing and can support long-term vagal tone improvement.

4. **Use Technology for Sound Therapy**: Many apps and online platforms offer sound therapy tools, including binaural beats, guided meditations, and nature sounds. Use them during times of stress or as part of your daily relaxation routine.

Conclusion

Music and sound are powerful tools for enhancing vagal tone, promoting relaxation, and supporting overall health. Whether through listening to music, chanting, singing, or participating in sound therapy sessions, sound can activate the vagus nerve and help restore balance to the body and mind. By incorporating sound practices into your daily routine, you can reduce stress, improve emotional regulation, and strengthen your parasympathetic nervous system, leading to better physical health and greater emotional resilience.

In the next chapter, we will explore how quality sleep plays a key role in vagal health and provide practical tips for improving sleep quality by activating the vagus nerve.

Chapter 12: The Vagus Nerve and Sleep

Sleep is one of the most fundamental processes in the body's restoration and healing. It is during sleep that the body performs many critical functions, such as tissue repair, memory consolidation, and the regulation of mood. One often overlooked, yet profoundly important, aspect of sleep is its connection to the vagus nerve. The vagus nerve plays a significant role in regulating the body's ability to rest and recover, and its activity can have a direct impact on the quality of sleep.

In this chapter, we will explore how the vagus nerve influences sleep, how poor vagal tone can disrupt sleep patterns, and practical strategies for improving sleep quality through the activation of the vagus nerve.

The Vagus Nerve's Role in Restorative Sleep

The vagus nerve is a key player in the parasympathetic nervous system, which is responsible for the "rest and digest" functions of the body. When the vagus nerve is activated, it promotes relaxation by slowing the heart rate, lowering blood pressure, and reducing overall stress. These physiological responses are essential for initiating and maintaining restorative sleep.

Heart rate variability (HRV), which is a marker of vagal tone, has been found to be closely linked to the quality of sleep. People with higher HRV—indicating better vagal tone—tend to experience deeper, more restful sleep. On the other hand, lower HRV is often associated with poor sleep quality, increased wakefulness during the night, and difficulty entering deeper stages of restorative sleep.

The vagus nerve's impact on sleep can be seen in how it interacts with the **autonomic nervous system (ANS)**. When the body is stressed, the sympathetic nervous system (the "fight or flight" response) becomes activated, which can make it difficult to fall asleep or stay asleep. By activating the vagus nerve, the parasympathetic nervous system is engaged, helping the body relax and prepare for sleep.

How to Improve Sleep Quality by Activating the Vagus Nerve

Now that we understand how the vagus nerve influences sleep, let's look at how we can activate it to improve the quality of our rest. By incorporating vagus nerve stimulation techniques into your bedtime routine, you can promote relaxation, lower stress levels, and create a sleep environment that encourages deep, restorative sleep.

Deep Breathing Exercises

Technique

Progressive Muscle Relaxation (PMR)

Technique

Mindfulness Meditation

Technique

Cold Exposure (or Cold Therapy)

Technique

Aromatherapy

Technique

Regular Sleep Schedule

Tip

Limit Stimulants Before Bed

Tip

Sleep Rituals for Enhanced Vagal Tone

Creating a bedtime routine that promotes vagal activation can signal to the body that it's time to rest and recover. Here's an example of a relaxing bedtime routine that supports vagus nerve activation:

- **60 minutes before bed**: Dim the lights and begin winding down by reducing screen time (avoid phones, computers, or TVs). You might want to listen to calming music, practice mindfulness, or engage in light reading.
- **30 minutes before bed**: Engage in deep breathing exercises, progressive muscle relaxation, or a short meditation session to activate the vagus nerve.
- **10 minutes before bed**: Use aromatherapy or cold exposure to further encourage relaxation.
- **Sleep environment**: Make sure your bedroom is cool, dark, and quiet, with a comfortable mattress and pillows. A sleep mask and blackout curtains can help enhance the environment for sleep.

Conclusion

The vagus nerve plays an essential role in the quality of your sleep, and by incorporating specific techniques into your routine, you can improve your sleep patterns and overall well-being. Practices like deep breathing, mindfulness, cold exposure, and aromatherapy can activate the vagus nerve, reduce stress, and promote a restful night's sleep. A regular sleep schedule, along with a calming pre-sleep ritual, is crucial for maintaining healthy vagal tone and ensuring that you wake up feeling refreshed and rejuvenated.

In the next chapter, we will explore the role of the vagus nerve in pain management and how stimulation of the vagus nerve can help alleviate chronic pain and improve overall recovery.

Chapter 13: The Vagus Nerve and Pain Management

Pain is one of the most common and debilitating experiences in human life. Whether chronic or acute, pain can have a profound impact on quality of life, mental health, and daily functioning. While traditional pain management strategies often focus on medication or physical therapies, an emerging approach is to utilize the body's own nervous system, particularly the vagus nerve, to modulate pain.

The vagus nerve, which is the longest cranial nerve in the body, plays a significant role in regulating the autonomic nervous system, including the processes that manage pain perception and inflammation. This chapter will explore the role of the vagus nerve in pain regulation, how stimulating the vagus nerve can help alleviate chronic pain, and practical methods to activate the vagus nerve for effective pain management.

The Vagus Nerve's Role in Pain Regulation

Pain is generally understood as a complex experience involving sensory input, emotional response, and the brain's interpretation of these signals. The autonomic nervous system (ANS), which includes the sympathetic and parasympathetic branches, is responsible for the body's responses to pain. The sympathetic nervous system is involved in the "fight or flight" response, which heightens the body's sensitivity to pain, while the parasympathetic nervous system, regulated by the vagus nerve, is responsible for calming and restoring balance to the body.

The vagus nerve, by promoting parasympathetic activity, plays a crucial role in dampening the body's pain response. It helps regulate inflammation, which is a key component of many chronic pain conditions, including rheumatoid arthritis, fibromyalgia, and inflammatory bowel diseases. By increasing vagal tone, the body can modulate pain perception and reduce the inflammatory processes that exacerbate pain.

Research has shown that **vagus nerve stimulation (VNS)**—a technique in which electrical impulses are delivered to the vagus nerve—can reduce pain and inflammation. This has led to its use in treating conditions such as chronic migraines, epilepsy, and even depression, where pain is a significant symptom. Vagus nerve stimulation is particularly effective in the treatment of pain that is resistant to conventional therapies, offering hope for those suffering from chronic, unresolved pain.

Using Vagus Stimulation to Alleviate Chronic Pain

Vagus nerve stimulation can be delivered in several ways, each varying in its intensity and method of application. While invasive VNS involves the implantation of a device that sends electrical impulses to the vagus nerve, there are non-invasive methods that are accessible to most people and can be practiced at home. These methods activate the vagus nerve and help modulate the body's pain response.

Deep Breathing and Diaphragmatic Breathing

Technique

Vagus Nerve Stimulation Devices

How it works

Acupressure and Acupuncture

- **How it works**: Acupuncture needles are strategically placed along the body's meridians to stimulate certain points that are thought to be linked to the vagus nerve. In acupressure, gentle pressure is applied to these same points, which can be performed at home.
- **Technique**: Consult with a licensed acupuncturist to ensure proper technique and treatment. You can also apply acupressure on yourself by gently massaging the specific points on your neck, wrists, or feet that correspond to pain relief.

Cold Exposure and Cryotherapy

- **How it works**: Cold therapy stimulates the vagus nerve by activating the parasympathetic nervous system. Cold showers, ice baths, or even applying a cold compress to the painful area can activate the vagus nerve and reduce the intensity of pain.
- **Technique**: Start by splashing your face with cold water or taking a short, cool shower. Gradually increase the duration of exposure or try applying ice packs to areas of inflammation for 10–15 minutes.

Meditation and Mindfulness

Technique

Non-Invasive Methods for Vagus Nerve Activation

In addition to the above methods, there are other ways to activate the vagus nerve and help with pain management:

Singing, Chanting, or Humming

Technique

Massage and Touch

Technique

Conclusion

Pain, whether acute or chronic, can be overwhelming, but by utilizing the vagus nerve's power to regulate pain responses, we can take a more holistic approach to pain management. Stimulating the vagus nerve through techniques such as deep breathing, mindfulness, cold exposure, and non-invasive devices can reduce pain, alleviate inflammation, and improve overall well-being.

In the next chapter, we will explore how the vagus nerve helps build a resilient nervous system, contributing to better mental and emotional health, and explore ways to increase vagal tone for greater resilience.

Chapter 14: Building a Resilient Nervous System with the Vagus Nerve

In today's fast-paced and high-stress world, building a resilient nervous system is more important than ever. A resilient nervous system can help us manage stress more effectively, recover from challenges faster, and maintain mental and emotional stability during times of adversity. The vagus nerve, often referred to as the "superhighway" of the autonomic nervous system, plays a crucial role in building this resilience. By optimizing vagal tone, you can enhance your body's ability to respond to stress in a healthy way, improving overall physical and mental health.

In this chapter, we will explore how the vagus nerve contributes to a resilient nervous system, the importance of increasing vagal tone, and practical strategies to build a stronger, more resilient body and mind.

Understanding the Autonomic Nervous System's Role in Health

To understand the vagus nerve's role in building resilience, it's essential to first explore the autonomic nervous system (ANS). The ANS is responsible for regulating many involuntary bodily functions, such as heart rate, digestion, and respiration. It consists of two main branches:

1. **The Sympathetic Nervous System (SNS)**: Often referred to as the "fight or flight" system, the SNS is responsible for preparing the body to respond to perceived threats. When activated, it increases heart rate, dilates the pupils, and releases stress hormones such as adrenaline, enabling the body to react quickly to danger.
2. **The Parasympathetic Nervous System (PNS)**: The PNS, which is regulated by the vagus nerve, is often referred to as the "rest and digest" system. It calms the body down after a stress response, slowing the heart rate, lowering blood pressure, and promoting relaxation and recovery.

The balance between the SNS and PNS is essential for maintaining optimal health. When the SNS is overactive, chronic stress and anxiety can result, leading to health issues such as hypertension, digestive problems, and burnout. In contrast, an underactive PNS can impair the body's ability to recover from stress, leaving you feeling fatigued and emotionally drained.

The vagus nerve acts as a bridge between these two systems. It helps to regulate the intensity of the stress response, and its activation promotes the calming effects of the PNS. When the vagus nerve is functioning optimally, it can help you bounce back from stressful situations more easily, leading to greater resilience.

Strategies for Increasing Vagal Tone for Greater Resilience

Vagal tone refers to the activity of the vagus nerve and its influence on the parasympathetic nervous system. Higher vagal tone is associated with better health outcomes, including lower stress levels, improved heart rate variability (HRV), and a stronger immune system. Low vagal tone, on the other hand, is linked to anxiety, depression, and an impaired ability to handle stress.

Fortunately, there are several ways to increase vagal tone and strengthen the parasympathetic response, leading to a more resilient nervous system. Here are some of the most effective strategies:

Breathing Techniques

Technique

diaphragmatic breathing

Physical Exercise

Exercise Tips

Meditation and Mindfulness

Practice Tip

Cold Exposure

Cold Exposure Tips

Positive Social Connections

Social Engagement Tips

Laughter

Laughter Tip

Building Mental Toughness and Emotional Balance

In addition to these physical practices, building mental toughness is a key part of creating a resilient nervous system. Mental toughness involves the ability to remain calm and focused under pressure, bounce back from adversity, and maintain a positive outlook. The vagus nerve plays a key role in emotional regulation, allowing you to manage negative emotions like fear, anger, and frustration more effectively.

Here are some techniques to build mental toughness and emotional balance:

1. **Cognitive Reframing**: This involves changing the way you think about stressful situations. Instead of focusing on the negative aspects, try to reframe challenges as opportunities for growth. By shifting your perspective, you can reduce stress and increase resilience.

2. **Gratitude Practice**: Practicing gratitude has been shown to improve emotional regulation, increase vagal tone, and enhance overall well-being. Each day, write down three things you're grateful for and reflect on how they contribute to your life. This simple practice can improve emotional balance and build resilience over time.

3. **Self-Compassion**: Practicing self-compassion involves treating yourself with kindness and understanding, particularly in times of struggle. Being gentle with yourself during difficult times can help you manage stress more effectively and support emotional resilience.

Conclusion

The vagus nerve plays a central role in building a resilient nervous system. By increasing vagal tone through practices such as deep breathing, physical exercise, mindfulness, and cold exposure, you can improve your ability to handle stress, recover from adversity, and maintain emotional balance. Strengthening the vagus nerve is not just about reducing stress; it's about creating a foundation of resilience that supports both your mental and physical health.

In the next chapter, we will explore the connection between the vagus nerve and emotional regulation, and how you can harness the power of the vagus nerve to manage negative emotions and improve emotional stability.

Chapter 15: The Vagus Nerve and Emotional Regulation

Emotions are a fundamental part of being human, influencing our thoughts, behaviors, and overall well-being. However, for many people, the experience of overwhelming or uncontrolled emotions can be debilitating. This is where the vagus nerve, with its powerful influence over the parasympathetic nervous system, plays a pivotal role. By understanding how the vagus nerve helps regulate emotional responses, we can unlock tools to improve emotional resilience, manage stress, and cultivate emotional stability.

In this chapter, we will explore how the vagus nerve helps regulate emotions, how vagal tone affects emotional health, and practical techniques to use the vagus nerve to enhance emotional regulation.

How the Vagus Nerve Controls Emotional Responses

The autonomic nervous system (ANS) plays a central role in the regulation of emotional responses, and the vagus nerve is a key component of this system. The ANS consists of two branches: the sympathetic nervous system (SNS), which triggers the "fight or flight" response, and the parasympathetic nervous system (PNS), which is primarily regulated by the vagus nerve and is responsible for the "rest and digest" response.

When the SNS is activated, our bodies prepare for action, typically in response to stress or perceived danger. This activation leads to increased heart rate, rapid breathing, heightened alertness, and a focus on survival. While this response is vital in short-term, high-stress situations, prolonged activation of the SNS can lead to chronic stress, anxiety, and emotional dysregulation.

On the other hand, the vagus nerve, which is the primary conduit for parasympathetic activity, acts as a counterbalance. When the vagus nerve is activated, it calms the body, slowing the heart rate, reducing blood pressure, and promoting relaxation. By promoting parasympathetic activity, the vagus nerve helps us return to a state of emotional balance after experiencing stress or overwhelming emotions.

This mechanism of calming down after emotional arousal is known as "vagal regulation," and it is essential for emotional well-being. A well-functioning vagus nerve allows us to respond to stressful situations more calmly and recover from emotional events more efficiently.

Vagal Tone and Emotional Stability

Vagal tone refers to the degree of activity of the vagus nerve and is often measured by heart rate variability (HRV), which refers to the variation in the time interval between heartbeats. Higher vagal tone is associated with greater emotional flexibility, resilience, and the ability to recover from stress. People with higher vagal tone are better able to shift between states of arousal and relaxation, which is a key component of emotional regulation.

Conversely, low vagal tone has been linked to several emotional challenges, including anxiety, depression, and difficulty managing stress. Low vagal tone may result in an overactive SNS response, which can lead to chronic feelings of tension, irritability, or emotional outbursts.

By improving vagal tone, you can enhance your emotional stability and improve your ability to cope with life's emotional ups and downs. Increased vagal tone has been shown to support better mood regulation, improved stress resilience, and enhanced emotional intelligence.

Techniques for Managing Negative Emotions Using the Vagus Nerve

Deep Breathing Exercises

Technique

diaphragmatic breathing

Mindfulness Meditation

Technique

mindfulness meditation

Progressive Muscle Relaxation (PMR)

Technique

Cold Exposure

Technique

Singing, Chanting, or Humming

Technique

Physical Exercise

Technique

Social Connection

Technique

Conclusion

The vagus nerve plays an integral role in regulating emotional responses, and by improving vagal tone, we can enhance our ability to manage emotions effectively. Techniques such as deep breathing, mindfulness, progressive muscle relaxation, cold exposure, singing, physical exercise, and positive social interactions all stimulate the vagus nerve and support emotional balance. By practicing these techniques regularly, you can cultivate a calm, centered, and resilient emotional state, better equipped to handle the challenges that life throws your way.

In the next chapter, we will explore how the vagus nerve affects heart health and how you can use vagal stimulation to improve cardiovascular function, further supporting your overall well-being.

Chapter 16: The Vagus Nerve and Your Heart

The connection between the vagus nerve and heart health is profound, influencing everything from heart rate to overall cardiovascular function. Understanding this relationship and learning how to stimulate the vagus nerve for heart health can provide significant benefits, not just in terms of physical health but also for emotional well-being. In this chapter, we will explore the fascinating link between the vagus nerve and the heart, how heart rate variability (HRV) serves as a marker of vagal tone, and how stimulating the vagus nerve can help maintain a healthy heart.

Heart Rate Variability and Vagal Tone

Heart rate variability (HRV) refers to the variation in time between consecutive heartbeats. A higher HRV is a sign of a well-functioning autonomic nervous system, where the parasympathetic system, regulated by the vagus nerve, can effectively counterbalance the sympathetic nervous system's "fight or flight" response.

HRV is considered a key indicator of overall health, and it plays a crucial role in cardiovascular health. Higher HRV is linked to improved cardiovascular function, reduced risk of heart disease, and better resilience to stress. Conversely, lower HRV is associated with a higher risk of cardiovascular problems, including hypertension, heart disease, and arrhythmias.

The vagus nerve plays a central role in regulating HRV by promoting the parasympathetic response, slowing down the heart rate, and allowing the body to enter a state of relaxation after stress. The more active the vagus nerve, the more variability there is in heart rate, and the better the heart can adapt to stressors.

How the Vagus Nerve Impacts Cardiovascular Health

The vagus nerve has several direct effects on the cardiovascular system that contribute to heart health:

1. **Slowing Heart Rate**: The vagus nerve helps slow the heart rate by signaling the heart's pacemaker, the sinoatrial node, to reduce its firing rate. This is particularly beneficial during times of stress or physical exertion, as it helps the body return to a state of calm and recovery.

2. **Lowering Blood Pressure**: Activation of the vagus nerve can help lower blood pressure by promoting vasodilation, or the relaxation of blood vessels. This helps to reduce the strain on the heart and circulatory system, decreasing the risk of hypertension.

3. **Reducing Inflammation**: Chronic inflammation is a significant risk factor for heart disease, contributing to the development of atherosclerosis (plaque buildup in the arteries). The vagus nerve helps regulate inflammation through the cholinergic anti-inflammatory pathway, which reduces the inflammatory response in the body, including in the heart and blood vessels.

4. **Supporting Heart Rate Recovery**: After physical exertion or stress, the vagus nerve helps the heart rate return to normal more quickly. This ability to recover rapidly is a sign of cardiovascular resilience and overall health.

5. **Preventing Arrhythmias**: The vagus nerve can help prevent abnormal heart rhythms (arrhythmias) by maintaining a healthy balance between the sympathetic and parasympathetic nervous systems. This helps to stabilize heart rhythm and reduce the risk of irregular heartbeats.

Given the significant role the vagus nerve plays in regulating cardiovascular function, finding ways to stimulate and optimize its activity can have a profound impact on heart health. Fortunately, there are several methods to increase vagal tone and improve cardiovascular function. Let's explore some of the most effective techniques for stimulating the vagus nerve to support heart health.

Deep Breathing and Diaphragmatic Breathing

Technique

diaphragmatic breathing

Exercise

Exercise Tip

Yoga and Meditation

- **Yoga Tip**: Incorporate practices such as **hatha yoga** or **restorative yoga** into your routine. Focus on deep breathing during each posture, and spend time in relaxation at the end of your session to activate the parasympathetic response.
- **Meditation Tip**: Practice mindfulness or **loving-kindness meditation**, which helps calm the mind and promote relaxation. Focus on your breath, allowing your body to relax with each inhale and exhale. Even 10-15 minutes per day can have a positive impact on vagal tone and heart health.

Cold Exposure

Cold Exposure Tip

cold showers

cold water immersion

Laughter

Laughter Tip

Massage

Massage Tip

Conclusion

The vagus nerve plays a central role in regulating heart function, from controlling heart rate to improving blood pressure and enhancing heart rate variability. By stimulating the vagus nerve through techniques such as deep breathing, exercise, yoga, cold exposure, and laughter, you can support cardiovascular health and improve overall well-being. In the next chapter, we will explore how the vagus nerve influences the immune system and how stimulating it can help reduce inflammation and enhance immune function.

Chapter 17: The Vagus Nerve and the Immune System

The immune system is the body's first line of defense against harmful pathogens, viruses, and bacteria. Its proper function is vital for health, yet the immune system is often compromised by chronic inflammation, stress, or poor lifestyle choices. Interestingly, the vagus nerve plays a crucial role in regulating immune responses and inflammation, offering a unique approach to enhancing immune function and protecting the body from disease. In this chapter, we will explore how the vagus nerve modulates the immune system, its influence on inflammation, and how you can leverage this connection to boost your immune health.

Vagus Nerve Modulation of Inflammation

Inflammation is a natural response to injury or infection, but when it becomes chronic, it can lead to a variety of health problems, including autoimmune diseases, heart disease, and even cancer. Chronic inflammation has been linked to many of the major health issues faced by modern society, making its regulation a critical aspect of long-term health.

The vagus nerve plays a key role in regulating the body's inflammatory response. It helps control inflammation through a mechanism known as the **cholinergic anti-inflammatory pathway**. This pathway is activated when the vagus nerve sends signals to the spleen, which then releases acetylcholine. Acetylcholine is a neurotransmitter that has been shown to inhibit the production of pro-inflammatory cytokines—proteins that promote inflammation—thereby reducing inflammation in the body.

This process is particularly significant in conditions where inflammation is a major concern, such as rheumatoid arthritis, inflammatory bowel disease, and cardiovascular disease. The vagus nerve essentially acts as a "brake" on the immune system, preventing it from becoming overactive and causing excessive inflammation.

Enhancing Immune Function Through Vagus Activation

By stimulating the vagus nerve, you can increase its activity and enhance the body's ability to regulate inflammation and immune responses. Research has shown that vagal nerve stimulation (VNS)—either through invasive techniques or non-invasive methods—can have significant effects on the immune system, improving immune function and helping to reduce chronic inflammation.

Here are a few ways to activate the vagus nerve and support your immune system:

Breathing Techniques

Technique

Cold Exposure

Cold Exposure Tip

Mindfulness and Meditation

Meditation Tip

Exercise

Exercise Tip

Massage

Massage Tip

Preventing Autoimmune Diseases and Inflammatory Conditions

The ability of the vagus nerve to regulate inflammation also plays a role in preventing autoimmune diseases and other chronic inflammatory conditions. In autoimmune diseases, the immune system mistakenly attacks the body's own tissues. Conditions like rheumatoid arthritis, lupus, and multiple sclerosis are characterized by chronic inflammation and immune dysfunction.

By stimulating the vagus nerve, you can help prevent this type of immune system overactivity. Research into **vagus nerve stimulation (VNS)** has shown promising results in treating conditions like rheumatoid arthritis, with patients experiencing significant reductions in inflammation and improvements in symptoms.

Additionally, the vagus nerve may help regulate the immune system's response to infections, potentially improving outcomes in cases of acute illness or infections. By supporting the vagus nerve's role in maintaining a balanced immune system, you can enhance the body's ability to fight off infections without triggering excessive inflammation.

The Role of Vagus Nerve Stimulation (VNS) in Autoimmune Disease

Vagus nerve stimulation (VNS) has emerged as a potential therapeutic option for autoimmune diseases and inflammatory conditions. VNS has been used experimentally to treat conditions like rheumatoid arthritis and inflammatory bowel disease (IBD), showing that direct stimulation of the vagus nerve can help reduce symptoms of these chronic conditions.

In some cases, VNS is administered using an implanted device that delivers electrical impulses to the vagus nerve. However, non-invasive methods such as deep breathing, meditation, and cold exposure can also activate the vagus nerve and provide similar benefits for inflammation and immune function, without the need for medical devices.

Conclusion

The vagus nerve plays an integral role in the regulation of the immune system and inflammation. By increasing vagal tone through lifestyle practices like deep breathing, meditation, cold exposure, and exercise, you can harness the power of the vagus nerve to reduce chronic inflammation, strengthen immune function, and prevent autoimmune diseases. This chapter highlights the importance of the vagus nerve as a regulatory mechanism for immune health, providing you with the tools to support a resilient immune system and enhance your overall health.

In the next chapter, we will explore how the vagus nerve influences gut health, a topic deeply interconnected with immune function, and how you can use vagal stimulation to support your digestive system.

Chapter 18: The Role of the Vagus Nerve in Gut Health

The connection between the brain and the gut has long been known, but recent research has highlighted the pivotal role of the vagus nerve in maintaining this connection. The vagus nerve is an essential pathway in the **gut-brain axis**, a bidirectional communication network that links the gut and the central nervous system. This relationship plays a vital role in regulating digestion, immune function, and emotional well-being. In this chapter, we will explore how the vagus nerve influences gut health and the ways in which you can leverage this knowledge to improve your digestive system and overall well-being.

The Gut-Brain Axis Explained

The **gut-brain axis** refers to the complex signaling system that connects the gut to the brain through neural, hormonal, and immune pathways. The vagus nerve serves as one of the primary communication routes between the gut and the brain. It carries signals from the gut to the brain and vice versa, allowing the body to maintain balance in digestion, immunity, and emotional health.

Approximately **90% of the communication** between the gut and the brain flows from the gut to the brain, rather than the other way around. This underlines the importance of gut health in influencing mood, cognition, and overall health. The vagus nerve plays a role in this communication, helping to regulate various functions such as:

- **Peristalsis**: The wave-like muscle contractions that move food through the digestive tract.
- **Enzyme secretion**: The release of digestive enzymes that help break down food for absorption.
- **Gut microbiota balance**: The vagus nerve influences the composition and activity of the gut microbiome, which is essential for digestion and immunity.

In essence, the vagus nerve helps the gut and the brain talk to each other, ensuring that the digestive system functions efficiently while maintaining the integrity of the body's overall health.

Vagal Stimulation to Improve Digestive Health

Vagal stimulation has been shown to have beneficial effects on gastrointestinal health. By activating the vagus nerve, you can promote the proper functioning of the digestive system, reduce inflammation, and improve gut motility. Some of the ways vagal stimulation enhances digestive health include:

- **Enhancing digestion**: Vagal activity promotes the secretion of digestive enzymes and bile, both of which are essential for breaking down food and absorbing nutrients. A well-functioning vagus nerve ensures that your digestive process operates smoothly and efficiently.
- **Improving gut motility**: Vagal stimulation encourages peristalsis, the muscular movements that propel food through the digestive system. It also helps maintain the balance between the muscles that contract and relax in the digestive tract, supporting healthy bowel movements and reducing symptoms like constipation or bloating.
- **Reducing gut inflammation**: Chronic inflammation in the gut is a hallmark of conditions like irritable bowel syndrome (IBS), Crohn's disease, and ulcerative colitis. The vagus nerve has anti-inflammatory effects, helping to regulate the immune response in the gut and reduce excessive inflammation. By improving vagal tone, you may be able to manage these conditions more effectively.
- **Modulating gut microbiota**: Recent studies have suggested that the vagus nerve can influence the composition and function of the gut microbiota, the trillions of microorganisms living in the digestive system. The vagus nerve helps to maintain a healthy balance of bacteria in the gut, which is essential for digestive function, immune health, and even mood regulation.

By incorporating practices that stimulate the vagus nerve, you can support your digestive system and foster a healthier gut-brain connection.

Healing the Gut with the Power of the Vagus Nerve

The health of the gut is intricately connected to overall well-being. When the vagus nerve is activated, it not only promotes digestion but also aids in healing and restoring the gut. The vagus nerve has shown therapeutic potential in conditions like **IBS, Crohn's disease**, and **leaky gut syndrome**, as it supports:

- **Gut barrier integrity**: The vagus nerve helps maintain the integrity of the gut lining, preventing "leaky gut"—a condition in which toxins and undigested food particles leak into the bloodstream. This dysfunction can trigger inflammation and immune responses, contributing to various chronic diseases. By enhancing vagal tone, you can support the gut's barrier function and reduce the risk of this condition.

- **Balancing the autonomic nervous system**: Chronic stress can alter the balance between the sympathetic and parasympathetic nervous systems, negatively affecting gut health. Stress-induced changes can lead to gut dysbiosis (imbalance of the gut microbiome), increased gut permeability, and even digestive disorders like acid reflux. Vagal stimulation helps bring balance to the autonomic nervous system, improving digestive function and lowering stress-induced gut symptoms.

- **Promoting gut healing**: For individuals suffering from gastrointestinal disorders or after a course of antibiotics that disrupts the gut microbiota, vagal stimulation can help accelerate gut healing. Practices such as deep breathing, meditation, and certain physical exercises can activate the vagus nerve and promote a healing environment in the gut.

Practical Tips for Vagal Stimulation to Support Gut Health

There are several ways to activate the vagus nerve and improve gut health through lifestyle changes and daily practices:

1. **Deep Breathing and Diaphragmatic Breathing**: As mentioned in earlier chapters, deep breathing exercises, especially diaphragmatic breathing, can activate the vagus nerve and reduce stress. To promote gut health, try incorporating a few minutes of deep breathing into your daily routine to enhance digestion and reduce gut inflammation.

2. **Cold Exposure**: Cold exposure, such as cold showers or ice baths, activates the vagus nerve and helps improve gut motility. If you're new to cold exposure, start with short bursts of cold water at the end of your regular shower. Over time, this practice can help regulate digestive processes and enhance gut health.

3. **Probiotics and Prebiotics**: The vagus nerve's influence on the microbiota is an important factor in gut health. Incorporating probiotics and prebiotics into your diet can support healthy gut bacteria. Foods like yogurt, kefir, fermented vegetables, and fiber-rich foods help create an optimal environment for beneficial bacteria, which can be enhanced by vagal activation.

4. **Mindfulness and Meditation**: Stress reduction practices, such as mindfulness meditation, have been shown to improve gut health by modulating the vagus nerve and reducing inflammation. Engaging in mindful eating practices can also improve digestion, as it encourages slow, relaxed eating, which is beneficial for gut health.

5. **Physical Exercise**: Regular physical activity, particularly aerobic exercise, helps stimulate the vagus nerve and supports healthy digestion. Walking, jogging, swimming, and yoga can help maintain gut motility and reduce the symptoms of digestive disorders.

Conclusion

The vagus nerve is an essential component of the gut-brain axis, directly influencing digestive health, gut motility, and inflammation. By stimulating the vagus nerve, you can improve digestion, reduce inflammation, and support the healing of the gut. Practices like deep breathing, cold exposure, meditation, and exercise can help maintain a healthy gut-brain connection and promote overall well-being.

In the next chapter, we will explore the role of the vagus nerve in aging, and how you can use vagal stimulation to slow down age-related decline in health and improve quality of life as you age.

Chapter 19: The Vagus Nerve in Aging

Aging is a natural process that brings many physiological changes to the body. As we age, we experience a gradual decline in various bodily functions, including the regulation of the autonomic nervous system (ANS), of which the vagus nerve plays a key role. The vagus nerve, often referred to as the "rest and digest" nerve, influences many essential functions such as heart rate, digestion, and immune function. In this chapter, we will explore how the vagus nerve changes with age, its role in maintaining health as we grow older, and how stimulating the vagus nerve can help prevent or even reverse age-related decline.

How Vagal Tone Changes with Age

Vagal tone refers to the level of activity or responsiveness of the vagus nerve. High vagal tone is associated with better overall health, including improved cardiovascular health, balanced emotions, and a well-functioning digestive system. Conversely, low vagal tone is often linked to an increased risk of chronic diseases, including heart disease, inflammation, and mental health disorders.

As we age, **vagal tone typically decreases**, which can contribute to a range of age-related health problems. Lower vagal tone has been shown to be a risk factor for conditions like:

- **Heart disease**: Low vagal tone is often associated with an increased heart rate and reduced heart rate variability (HRV), both of which are markers of poor cardiovascular health.
- **Chronic inflammation**: The vagus nerve has anti-inflammatory properties, and reduced vagal activity can lead to higher levels of systemic inflammation, which is linked to aging-related diseases such as arthritis, diabetes, and neurodegenerative conditions.
- **Cognitive decline**: The vagus nerve also plays a role in brain health. Decreased vagal tone can contribute to cognitive decline and conditions like Alzheimer's disease.
- **Weakened immune system**: The vagus nerve helps regulate immune responses. As vagal tone decreases with age, the immune system may become less efficient, increasing the susceptibility to infections and other health issues.

Understanding these changes is crucial, as maintaining or improving vagal tone can significantly impact the aging process and promote a healthier, more vibrant life.

Preventing Age-Related Decline through Vagal Stimulation

While aging is inevitable, we do not have to accept the associated decline in health. One of the most effective ways to counteract these age-related changes is through **vagal nerve stimulation** (VNS). Stimulating the vagus nerve has been shown to have wide-ranging benefits for the body and brain, and it can play a key role in slowing down or even reversing certain aspects of aging.

There are several approaches to stimulating the vagus nerve, and each of these methods can help improve your overall health and vitality:

1. **Breathing Exercises**: Slow, deep breathing stimulates the vagus nerve and helps to increase vagal tone. Techniques such as diaphragmatic breathing, box breathing, and alternate nostril breathing activate the parasympathetic nervous system, promoting relaxation and improving heart rate variability. These simple exercises can be done daily to counteract the effects of aging on the cardiovascular system.

2. **Physical Exercise**: Regular physical activity, particularly aerobic exercise, has been shown to increase vagal tone and improve heart rate variability. Cardiovascular exercises such as walking, jogging, swimming, or cycling can strengthen the heart, boost circulation, and enhance the functioning of the vagus nerve. Exercise also helps reduce chronic inflammation, which is one of the main contributors to age-related diseases.

3. **Cold Exposure**: Exposure to cold, such as cold showers or ice baths, can stimulate the vagus nerve and improve vagal tone. This method has been linked to enhanced cardiovascular health, improved immune function, and reduced inflammation. Cold exposure activates the parasympathetic nervous system, helping to balance out the effects of the sympathetic nervous system, which tends to dominate during stress.

4. **Meditation and Mindfulness**: Practices like mindfulness meditation and yoga have been shown to improve vagal tone by promoting relaxation and reducing stress. These practices activate the vagus nerve, enhancing its ability to regulate physiological functions. Meditation, particularly when focused on deep, slow breathing, can help restore balance to the autonomic nervous system and slow down the aging process.

5. **Diet and Nutrition**: A healthy diet that supports the nervous system and reduces inflammation can also help improve vagal tone. Foods rich in omega-3 fatty acids, antioxidants, and anti-inflammatory compounds support brain and heart health, reduce oxidative stress, and help maintain a healthy gut-brain axis. Probiotics, prebiotics, and fermented foods are also beneficial for gut health and can indirectly support vagal activity.

6. **Vagus Nerve Stimulation Devices**: In more advanced cases, medical devices designed to stimulate the vagus nerve can be used. These devices are typically implanted under the skin and deliver electrical pulses to the vagus nerve to treat conditions like epilepsy and depression. Recent research has also explored the use of non-invasive transcutaneous VNS devices, which can be used at home to stimulate the vagus nerve and improve health outcomes.

Reversing Age-Related Illnesses Using the Vagus Nerve

Beyond preventing decline, stimulating the vagus nerve may help **reverse certain age-related conditions**. Here's how vagal stimulation can support the treatment and management of common age-related ailments:

1. **Cardiovascular Health**: As mentioned, low vagal tone is associated with an increased risk of heart disease. By stimulating the vagus nerve, you can improve heart rate variability, lower blood pressure, and reduce the risk of developing cardiovascular conditions such as hypertension, arrhythmias, and heart attacks.

2. **Cognitive Decline and Neurodegenerative Diseases**: The vagus nerve is involved in brain health by promoting neuroplasticity and reducing inflammation. Research has shown that vagus nerve stimulation can enhance memory, improve cognitive function, and even help slow the progression of neurodegenerative diseases like Alzheimer's and Parkinson's disease.

3. **Chronic Inflammation**: As we age, chronic low-level inflammation becomes more prevalent. This "inflammaging" is linked to several age-related diseases, including arthritis, diabetes, and cancer. The vagus nerve has powerful anti-inflammatory effects, and activating it can reduce systemic inflammation, improving overall health and quality of life.

4. **Depression and Anxiety**: Mental health issues, such as depression and anxiety, are common among older adults. Vagal stimulation has been shown to improve mood and emotional stability by regulating the stress response and promoting the release of feel-good hormones like serotonin. By improving vagal tone, you may be able to manage stress and anxiety more effectively and reduce the risk of depression.

The vagus nerve is a powerful tool in the fight against the physical and cognitive decline that accompanies aging. By integrating practices that stimulate the vagus nerve into your daily routine, you can not only slow down the aging process but also enhance your vitality and well-being. The key is to take a holistic approach that includes:

- **Consistent physical activity** to enhance cardiovascular and brain health.
- **Mindfulness practices** to reduce stress and improve emotional stability.
- **Healthy eating** to support brain, heart, and gut health.
- **Cold exposure** and **vagus nerve stimulation devices** as adjunct therapies for more profound health improvements.

By focusing on maintaining or increasing vagal tone, you can support a healthier, more vibrant aging process.

Conclusion

The vagus nerve plays a central role in the aging process. As vagal tone decreases with age, various health issues, including cardiovascular disease, cognitive decline, and chronic inflammation, can emerge. However, by stimulating the vagus nerve through lifestyle changes such as deep breathing, exercise, meditation, and proper nutrition, you can counteract these effects and enhance your quality of life.

In the next chapter, we will explore the concept of biohacking the vagus nerve, using advanced techniques and technologies to further optimize its function for long-term health and longevity.

Chapter 20: Biohacking the Vagus Nerve

In recent years, the concept of biohacking has gained significant attention. The idea of taking control of our biology—improving, enhancing, or optimizing our health and physical function through conscious lifestyle changes—has become a popular approach to living longer, healthier lives. One area where biohacking can have a powerful impact is through the optimization of the vagus nerve. By intentionally stimulating and strengthening the vagus nerve, individuals can improve their overall health, enhance their brain function, and mitigate the effects of stress, inflammation, and even aging.

In this chapter, we will explore the concept of biohacking the vagus nerve, detailing both advanced techniques and wearable technologies that can help optimize vagal function. Whether through lifestyle adjustments, innovative tools, or the latest cutting-edge technologies, there are numerous ways to take control of your vagus nerve and tap into its full potential.

Advanced Techniques for Vagus Nerve Optimization

The vagus nerve offers a variety of health benefits when its function is optimized. Beyond the basic techniques such as deep breathing, meditation, and exercise, there are more advanced methods that specifically target vagal tone and stimulate its activity. These techniques can be used to optimize vagus nerve performance for better physical health, emotional balance, and mental clarity.

1. **Vagus Nerve Stimulation (VNS) Therapy**:

    Vagus nerve stimulation (VNS) is a medically approved treatment for conditions such as epilepsy and depression, involving the implantation of a device that delivers electrical impulses to the vagus nerve. This therapy has been studied and found to have profound effects on mood regulation, brain health, and inflammation control. Recent developments have led to the creation of **non-invasive VNS devices**, which use electrical impulses delivered through the skin, typically around the ear or neck area. These devices can be worn at home and offer an easy, non-invasive way to activate the vagus nerve, enhancing vagal tone without the need for surgery. These devices are used to treat conditions like depression, anxiety, and chronic pain, with growing evidence suggesting their broader health benefits. **How it works**: VNS works by sending electrical pulses through the vagus nerve, stimulating the parasympathetic nervous system and promoting a calming effect throughout the body. This stimulation helps to reduce inflammation, improve heart rate variability (HRV), and encourage better mental clarity and mood stability. Many individuals use VNS to manage stress, improve sleep, and even reduce the symptoms of chronic inflammatory conditions like arthritis.

2. **Transcutaneous Auricular Vagus Nerve Stimulation (taVNS):**

   This non-invasive technique involves stimulating the vagus nerve via electrodes placed on the ear. Research suggests that stimulating the auricular branch of the vagus nerve has a variety of therapeutic benefits, including improved mood regulation, reduced anxiety, and enhanced cognitive function. **How it works**: By placing electrodes on the ear, taVNS stimulates the auricular branch of the vagus nerve, which is accessible via the outer ear. This stimulation is known to activate brain regions involved in emotional regulation, pain control, and cognitive function, providing a relatively easy way to biohack the vagus nerve. Devices for taVNS are portable, allowing users to receive therapy from the comfort of their own homes.

3. **Breathing Techniques Enhanced by Biofeedback**:

    While deep breathing exercises can stimulate the vagus nerve naturally, biofeedback devices take this process to the next level. These devices track physiological functions like heart rate variability (HRV) and provide real-time feedback, helping individuals improve their breathing techniques and enhance vagal tone more effectively. **How it works**: Biofeedback devices measure your heart rate and provide visual or auditory signals that guide your breathing to increase HRV, which is a direct measure of vagal tone. When you breathe deeply and slowly, your heart rate will naturally slow down, signaling an increase in parasympathetic nervous system activity. Biofeedback tools help you learn how to control this process and optimize your vagal tone, leading to better stress resilience, relaxation, and emotional regulation.

Wearables and Gadgets to Enhance Vagal Tone

In addition to the techniques mentioned above, there are a growing number of wearables and gadgets designed to stimulate and optimize vagal tone. These devices are part of the growing trend in health tech, where biohacking intersects with modern technology. They help users to engage with the autonomic nervous system in real-time, giving individuals more control over their health.

1. **Heart Rate Variability (HRV) Monitors**:

   HRV is a direct measure of vagal tone, and enhancing HRV is one of the most effective ways to biohack the vagus nerve. HRV monitors are wearable devices that track the time variation between heartbeats. A higher HRV typically indicates a healthier autonomic nervous system with a dominant parasympathetic (vagal) influence. **How it works**: These devices typically use sensors placed on the chest, wrist, or finger to monitor the intervals between heartbeats. By tracking HRV, users can assess the effectiveness of their vagus nerve stimulation techniques. When HRV increases, it's a sign that vagal tone is improving, which can be achieved through practices like deep breathing, physical activity, and meditation.

2. **Neurostimulation Devices**:

   Some biohacking enthusiasts use wearable neurostimulation devices that deliver targeted electrical pulses to the body, promoting vagal activation and reducing stress levels. These devices are designed to enhance vagal tone through external stimulation, often using low-level electrical currents. **How it works**: These devices work by applying gentle electrical impulses to the skin, targeting the vagus nerve. Over time, regular use of neurostimulation devices can help regulate inflammation, improve cardiovascular health, and boost cognitive function. Some wearable devices use specific waveforms and frequencies of stimulation that are optimized for vagus nerve activation.

3. **Wearable Meditation and Relaxation Tools**:

    Devices that combine mindfulness training with technology are increasingly popular for enhancing vagal tone. These tools often guide users through meditative practices, such as deep breathing, while providing real-time biofeedback to optimize their autonomic nervous system regulation. **How it works**: Wearable devices like guided breathwork apps or meditation headbands track your brainwaves, heart rate, and breathing patterns during meditation. These devices provide feedback to ensure you're breathing deeply and effectively, which helps stimulate the vagus nerve. Over time, regular use of these tools can lead to sustained increases in vagal tone.

The Future of Vagus Nerve Stimulation

As research continues into the complex role of the vagus nerve in health, the potential for biohacking and vagal optimization continues to expand. Future developments may bring even more innovative devices and technologies to market, enhancing our ability to regulate the autonomic nervous system and maintain overall health.

1. **Advances in Non-Invasive Vagus Nerve Stimulation**:

    As technology progresses, we can expect more sophisticated, user-friendly, and non-invasive VNS devices that allow individuals to safely stimulate their vagus nerve at home. These devices may become more widely accessible for the management of mental health, chronic pain, and other conditions.

2. **Artificial Intelligence (AI) and Biohacking**:

    AI could revolutionize the way we understand and optimize the vagus nerve. By using machine learning algorithms, we may be able to develop more personalized vagus nerve stimulation protocols that adapt in real-time to an individual's physiological responses, maximizing vagal tone and improving health outcomes.

3. **Genetic Modulation of Vagal Tone**:

    Future advancements might allow for genetic interventions that enhance the function of the vagus nerve. This could involve gene therapies designed to increase the responsiveness of the vagus nerve, leading to more effective regulation of the autonomic nervous system and enhanced health over the course of one's life.

Conclusion

Biohacking the vagus nerve is an exciting frontier in the realm of health optimization. Through advanced techniques like vagus nerve stimulation, wearable devices, and lifestyle modifications, it is now possible to enhance vagal tone and improve physical, emotional, and cognitive health. Whether you are looking to alleviate stress, improve cardiovascular function, or increase resilience against aging, biohacking the vagus nerve provides powerful tools to achieve these goals. As the science and technology around vagus nerve optimization evolve, the potential benefits are vast, and the future of health may be largely shaped by our ability to harness the power of the vagus nerve.

Chapter 21: Managing Stress with the Vagus Nerve

Stress is a natural response to perceived challenges, but when it becomes chronic, it can wreak havoc on our physical, emotional, and mental health. The autonomic nervous system, and particularly the vagus nerve, plays a key role in how we manage stress and maintain balance. Understanding how the vagus nerve helps regulate stress responses and learning how to harness its power can significantly improve our stress resilience, leading to a more peaceful, healthy, and productive life.

In this chapter, we will explore how the vagus nerve interacts with the body's stress response and provide practical strategies for managing stress through vagal stimulation. These strategies are designed to help you activate the parasympathetic nervous system, which is responsible for rest, digestion, and recovery, while reducing the impact of the fight-or-flight response triggered by the sympathetic nervous system.

The Stress Response and Vagal Dysfunction

To understand how the vagus nerve helps manage stress, it's essential to grasp how the stress response works in the body. When you face a stressor—whether physical or emotional—your body activates the sympathetic nervous system, triggering the fight-or-flight response. This response includes increased heart rate, heightened alertness, and the release of stress hormones like cortisol and adrenaline, all of which prepare your body to confront the threat.

While this response is helpful in short bursts, chronic stress can lead to negative health outcomes such as anxiety, heart disease, digestive issues, and mental fatigue. The vagus nerve, as part of the parasympathetic nervous system, helps to "shut off" the stress response by promoting relaxation and recovery.

However, chronic stress, poor lifestyle habits, and certain medical conditions can impair vagal function, leading to a reduced ability to regulate the stress response. Low vagal tone is associated with higher levels of stress, inflammation, and susceptibility to mental health issues. By improving vagal tone, we can help the body return to balance after stress and cultivate greater resilience over time.

Practical Strategies to Manage Stress through Vagal Stimulation

The good news is that you can actively improve your vagal tone and reduce stress through several practical techniques. These strategies help stimulate the vagus nerve, activating the parasympathetic nervous system and allowing the body to recover more efficiently from stress.

Deep Breathing Exercises

How to do it:

- Find a quiet, comfortable place to sit or lie down.
- Place one hand on your chest and the other on your abdomen.
- Take a slow, deep breath through your nose, allowing your abdomen to expand as your diaphragm moves downward.
- Exhale slowly through your mouth, letting go of tension as you breathe out.
- Aim for a slow, steady breathing rate of about 5–6 breaths per minute (inhale for a count of 4, exhale for a count of 6). Practicing this deep breathing technique for just 5–10 minutes a day can significantly lower stress and improve vagal tone.

Meditation and Mindfulness

How to do it:

- Sit comfortably with your spine straight and close your eyes.
- Focus on your breath or a specific word or mantra, gently bringing your attention back to your chosen point of focus whenever distractions arise.
- Practice mindfulness by observing any thoughts or feelings without judgment, simply letting them pass like clouds in the sky. Research has shown that regular meditation can increase vagal tone, reduce cortisol levels, and enhance overall stress resilience. Even just a few minutes a day can yield noticeable benefits.

Cold Exposure

How to do it:

- Gradually incorporate cold exposure into your routine. Start with a few seconds of cold water at the end of your shower and increase the duration as your body adapts.
- If you prefer, splash cold water on your face, particularly the area around the eyes and cheeks, to activate the vagus nerve. The shock from cold exposure causes an immediate increase in vagal tone, which helps reduce the stress response, lower heart rate, and promote relaxation.

Yoga and Tai Chi

How to do it:

- Begin with gentle yoga or tai chi classes, focusing on smooth, deliberate movements and deep breathing.
- Incorporate poses like child's pose, legs up the wall, or savasana, which are particularly calming and help stimulate the vagus nerve.
- Practice these activities regularly to build a routine that helps manage stress and improve overall vagal tone. Yoga and tai chi not only reduce stress but also improve flexibility, balance, and mental clarity, making them ideal practices for managing both physical and emotional tension.

Social Connection and Laughter

How to do it:

- Spend time with loved ones, engage in meaningful conversations, and laugh together.
- Watch a funny movie or participate in activities that make you smile and laugh.
- Aim to nurture relationships that provide emotional support and foster a sense of belonging. Laughter has been shown to stimulate the vagus nerve and lower levels of stress hormones, enhancing mood and promoting a state of calm.

Progressive Muscle Relaxation (PMR)

How to do it:

- Find a quiet space and sit or lie down comfortably.
- Start by tensing the muscles in your toes for 5-10 seconds, then relax them.
- Move up through your body, tensing and relaxing each muscle group (calves, thighs, abdomen, chest, arms, and face).
- Focus on the sensation of relaxation as you release tension from each muscle group. PMR helps you reconnect with your body, release stress, and activate the parasympathetic nervous system for a calming effect.

Creating a Stress-Free Lifestyle with Vagus Nerve Mastery

Managing stress is not just about using specific techniques in the moment; it's about cultivating a lifestyle that supports vagal health and reduces overall stress levels. Incorporating the strategies outlined in this chapter into your daily routine can help you build a resilient nervous system and enhance your capacity to handle stress effectively.

By prioritizing practices that activate the vagus nerve, you are strengthening your body's natural ability to recover from stress and remain balanced in the face of life's challenges. Over time, you'll notice an improved ability to manage emotional triggers, greater relaxation, and an increased sense of well-being. Ultimately, mastering your vagus nerve will empower you to lead a more calm, focused, and peaceful life.

Chapter 22: The Vagus Nerve and Cognitive Function

The connection between the vagus nerve and cognitive function is a fascinating area of study. This chapter explores how the vagus nerve influences brain health, memory, focus, and cognitive abilities. By understanding the mechanisms through which the vagus nerve supports brain health, you can implement practical strategies to optimize cognitive function and enhance mental clarity.

The Vagus Nerve and Brain Health

The vagus nerve plays a key role in the communication between the brain and body. As one of the longest nerves in the body, it has a direct influence on the brain's regulation of various functions, including emotional responses, stress levels, and even memory. The vagus nerve's ability to modulate brain activity is critical for maintaining optimal cognitive function and emotional well-being.

Through its connection to the parasympathetic nervous system, the vagus nerve helps regulate brain regions associated with learning, attention, and emotional regulation. By reducing stress and inflammation, it enables the brain to function efficiently and allows for enhanced memory retention and concentration.

Moreover, the vagus nerve has been linked to neuroplasticity, the brain's ability to adapt and form new neural connections. Vagal stimulation can enhance brain resilience, increase the capacity for learning, and support cognitive repair, particularly in those dealing with cognitive decline, such as in aging or neurodegenerative diseases.

Enhancing Memory, Focus, and Brain Health with Vagal Stimulation

Studies have shown that stimulating the vagus nerve can have a profound effect on brain function, particularly in areas responsible for memory and concentration. By increasing heart rate variability (HRV) and lowering stress levels, vagal stimulation promotes a calm, alert mental state conducive to focus and memory retention.

Vagal stimulation for brain health:

- **Neurogenesis:** Vagal nerve activation can stimulate the growth of new neurons, particularly in the hippocampus, which plays a key role in memory formation and cognitive processing.
- **Reduced stress:** Chronic stress inhibits cognitive function, but vagus nerve stimulation helps lower stress hormones like cortisol, protecting the brain from long-term damage.
- **Improved circulation:** Vagal activation improves blood flow to the brain, providing the necessary nutrients and oxygen for optimal brain function.

How to Stimulate the Vagus Nerve for Cognitive Enhancement:

Deep Breathing Exercises:

How to do it:

- Sit comfortably in a chair or on the floor, ensuring your spine is straight.
- Close your eyes and take a slow, deep breath through your nose, filling your belly first, then your chest. Inhale for a count of four.
- Hold the breath for a moment, then exhale slowly and steadily for a count of six.
- Repeat for five to ten minutes, allowing your mind to clear and your body to relax. Practicing this deep breathing exercise regularly can help improve mental clarity and reduce mental fatigue.

Meditation and Mindfulness:

How to do it:

- Start by sitting in a quiet space with your eyes closed.
- Focus on your breath or a specific sound, and gently bring your attention back to the present moment when distractions arise.
- You can also try mindfulness meditation techniques like "body scanning," where you focus on each part of your body to increase awareness and calm the mind. This practice not only helps reduce stress but also enhances attention and memory, as it trains the brain to focus on the present moment and improve cognitive performance.

Exercise and Vagal Stimulation:

How to do it:

- Engage in aerobic exercises like walking, jogging, or swimming. Aim for at least 30 minutes of moderate exercise three to five times a week.
- Yoga and tai chi, which combine gentle movement with deep breathing, also stimulate the vagus nerve and improve brain health. Consistent exercise has been linked to better memory, improved attention span, and a decreased risk of cognitive decline with age.

Cold Exposure:

How to do it:

- Incorporate cold showers at the end of your regular shower or take a brief ice bath.
- If this feels too intense, start with splashing cold water on your face or placing an ice pack on the back of your neck for 30 seconds to one minute. Over time, cold exposure can help improve cognitive function by reducing brain fog and enhancing mental sharpness.

Nutrition for Cognitive Health:

Foods to consider:

- **Omega-3 fatty acids:** Found in fatty fish like salmon, walnuts, and flaxseeds, omega-3s support brain health and improve cognitive function.
- **Antioxidants:** Blueberries, dark chocolate, and leafy greens help protect the brain from oxidative stress and support memory and learning.
- **Probiotic-rich foods:** Fermented foods like yogurt, kimchi, and kefir promote gut health, which in turn supports brain health via the gut-brain axis.

Social Interaction and Cognitive Enhancement:

How to do it:

- Spend quality time with family, friends, or pets. Engaging in stimulating conversations and social activities can promote cognitive health and emotional well-being.
- Volunteer, join clubs, or participate in group activities to enhance social interaction and reduce feelings of isolation.

The Role of the Vagus Nerve in Learning and Cognition

The vagus nerve is also deeply involved in the process of learning. By stimulating this nerve, you can enhance your ability to retain information, focus on tasks, and improve problem-solving skills. In the classroom or at work, implementing vagal-stimulating techniques can help you absorb and recall information more effectively.

As vagal stimulation reduces the stress response, it allows the brain to focus more clearly, retain new information, and approach complex tasks with a calm, organized mindset.

Tips for Enhancing Cognitive Performance

- **Prioritize sleep:** Quality sleep is crucial for brain health. It consolidates memory, facilitates learning, and restores cognitive function.
- **Stay mentally active:** Engage in brain exercises like puzzles, reading, or learning a new skill to keep the brain sharp.
- **Practice mindfulness:** Regular mindfulness practices reduce stress and improve mental clarity, attention, and decision-making skills.

Conclusion

Mastering the vagus nerve is one of the most effective ways to improve cognitive function, enhance memory, and boost mental clarity. By using the techniques outlined in this chapter—breathing exercises, meditation, exercise, cold exposure, and proper nutrition—you can activate the vagus nerve to support brain health and optimize cognitive performance. As you continue to integrate these practices into your daily life, you will find that your ability to focus, learn, and retain information improves, helping you become more productive, sharp, and mentally resilient.

Chapter 23: Using the Vagus Nerve for Personal Growth

The vagus nerve, often referred to as the "wandering nerve," has a profound impact on many aspects of human health and well-being. Beyond its role in physical health, the vagus nerve can be harnessed for personal growth, allowing individuals to enhance emotional intelligence, overcome limiting beliefs, and embark on transformative journeys. This chapter will explore the powerful connection between the vagus nerve and personal development, providing tools and techniques for using the vagus nerve to unlock your fullest potential.

Building Emotional Intelligence with Vagus Nerve Activation

Emotional intelligence (EQ) is the ability to recognize, understand, and manage our own emotions, as well as the emotions of others. High EQ is associated with better decision-making, stronger relationships, and greater overall well-being. The vagus nerve plays a pivotal role in emotional regulation, stress management, and the ability to stay calm and balanced under pressure—all essential components of emotional intelligence.

When vagal tone is strong, the body is better able to manage emotional reactions, reducing the likelihood of overreaction and fostering resilience. By stimulating the vagus nerve, we can improve our ability to be emotionally aware and regulate our responses in challenging situations.

Vagal Stimulation for Emotional Regulation:

- **Deep Breathing:** Deep, diaphragmatic breathing is one of the most effective ways to activate the vagus nerve and regulate emotions. By slowing the breath, we signal to the brain that it is time to relax, enabling emotional stability and clarity of thought.
- **Meditation:** Mindfulness and meditation practices that focus on the breath or body can strengthen the vagus nerve and enhance emotional awareness. These practices help you become more present, which is essential for responding thoughtfully to emotional triggers.

Practical Exercises:

- **Body Scan Meditation:** Start by focusing on your breath, and then mentally scan your body from head to toe, noticing any areas of tension or discomfort. Gently release any tension you find. This exercise helps to ground you in the present moment and activates the vagus nerve, which can improve emotional regulation.
- **Mindful Listening:** Practice being fully present when interacting with others. Focus on their words and emotions, and notice how your own emotional responses are triggered. By being mindful of your emotions and bodily sensations, you activate the vagus nerve, fostering greater emotional intelligence.

Overcoming Limiting Beliefs and Negative Thought Patterns

Limiting beliefs are those deep-seated thoughts that tell us we are not capable, worthy, or deserving of success and happiness. These beliefs can be rooted in past experiences or societal conditioning, and they often hold us back from realizing our full potential. The vagus nerve plays a significant role in overcoming limiting beliefs by influencing the way we process emotions and experiences.

By strengthening the vagus nerve, we can enhance the parasympathetic nervous system's ability to create a sense of calm, reducing anxiety and fear. This allows us to confront and reframe negative thought patterns, ultimately helping us to replace them with more empowering beliefs.

The Role of Vagus Stimulation in Reframing Beliefs:

- **Stress Reduction:** When we activate the vagus nerve, we engage the parasympathetic nervous system, reducing the stress and anxiety that often accompany negative thought patterns. This state of relaxation helps us approach challenges from a place of calm and clarity, making it easier to confront and challenge limiting beliefs.
- **Positive Reframing:** Vagus nerve activation can create a state of mental openness, allowing us to reframe negative beliefs and replace them with more constructive thoughts. When we feel safe and grounded, we are better equipped to challenge beliefs that no longer serve us.

Practical Exercises:

- **Affirmations and Vagal Activation:** Pair affirmations with vagal stimulation techniques. For example, while practicing deep breathing or mindfulness, repeat positive affirmations such as "I am capable of achieving my goals" or "I am worthy of success." The combination of these practices strengthens both your neural pathways and your belief system.
- **Visualization:** Visualize a specific scenario in which you previously felt limited by fear or self-doubt. As you engage in deep breathing or mindfulness, imagine yourself successfully navigating the situation. Visualizing positive outcomes while engaging the vagus nerve helps to reframe negative beliefs and increase self-confidence.

How to Use Vagal Techniques for Personal Transformation

Personal transformation involves the process of growing beyond old patterns of thought, behavior, and emotion. By utilizing vagal stimulation techniques, we can create a more supportive internal environment that nurtures transformation. These practices help us break free from old habits and step into our highest potential.

Steps to Personal Transformation through the Vagus Nerve:

1. **Activate the Vagus Nerve Regularly:** The more you activate the vagus nerve through deep breathing, meditation, and other techniques, the more it becomes a part of your daily routine. This consistent practice supports emotional regulation, resilience, and openness to new experiences, which are crucial for personal growth.

2. **Cultivate a Growth Mindset:** The vagus nerve helps regulate the stress response, allowing you to remain calm and focused when faced with challenges. This calm state encourages a growth mindset—seeing obstacles as opportunities for learning and growth. Embrace challenges, knowing that you have the tools to navigate them.

3. **Set Clear Intentions:** Transformation begins with clarity. Define your goals and intentions, and use vagal activation techniques to stay grounded and aligned with your purpose. The calm state fostered by vagus nerve activation enables you to remain focused on your goals and to remain open to new opportunities.

Practical Exercises:

- **Journaling and Reflection:** Set aside time each day to reflect on your progress and intentions. Write down your thoughts, feelings, and experiences with vagal stimulation practices. Journaling helps solidify new beliefs and behaviors and allows you to track your transformation.
- **Setting Intentions with Vagal Activation:** Before embarking on a new goal or challenge, take a few moments to breathe deeply and activate your vagus nerve. While in this calm, focused state, set clear intentions and visualize your success. This practice aligns your mind, body, and spirit toward positive transformation.

Conclusion

Mastering the vagus nerve offers a powerful tool for personal growth, emotional intelligence, and overcoming limiting beliefs. By incorporating vagal stimulation techniques into your daily life, you can cultivate resilience, emotional stability, and a growth mindset. These practices empower you to break free from old patterns and step into your highest potential. Whether you seek to improve your relationships, enhance your professional life, or experience greater emotional freedom, the vagus nerve holds the key to unlocking transformative growth.

Chapter 24: The Vagus Nerve in Practice: Real-World Applications

Understanding the theoretical aspects of the vagus nerve and its health benefits is important, but applying that knowledge in real life is where true transformation happens. This chapter will focus on the practical integration of vagus nerve techniques into daily life, share real-world examples of people who have successfully harnessed the power of the vagus nerve, and guide you in creating a personalized plan to master your vagal health.

Integrating Vagus Nerve Techniques into Daily Life

While many of the techniques to stimulate the vagus nerve—such as deep breathing, mindfulness, cold exposure, and physical activity—are simple, consistency is key. Incorporating these practices into your routine in a way that feels natural and sustainable can yield profound benefits in the long term.

Here are a few ways to integrate vagus nerve techniques into your daily activities:

1. Morning Routine: Starting the Day with Vagal Activation

- **Deep Breathing:** Upon waking up, spend a few minutes focusing on deep breathing or diaphragmatic breathing. This can help activate the parasympathetic nervous system and set a calm tone for the day ahead.
- **Cold Exposure:** Consider incorporating a cold shower or a brief splash of cold water to the face as part of your morning routine. This invigorates the vagus nerve and boosts energy levels for the day.
- **Mindfulness Moment:** Take a moment of stillness to meditate or simply check in with how you're feeling. A few minutes of mindfulness can increase your awareness and improve emotional regulation throughout the day.

2. During the Workday: Incorporating Stress-Reduction Techniques

- **Midday Break for Breathing Exercises:** If you experience stress or mental fatigue during the workday, take a short break to practice deep breathing. This helps maintain a steady focus and regulate your emotions.
- **Mindful Movement:** Take short walks throughout the day, particularly outside. Physical movement encourages vagal tone, and the outdoor environment can provide a calming, grounding effect.
- **Micro-Meditation:** Even just 3 to 5 minutes of focused breathing or mindfulness can reset your nervous system and help you refocus during a busy day.

3. Evening Routine: Preparing for Restful Sleep

- **Vagus Nerve Stimulation for Better Sleep:** Engage in calming practices such as diaphragmatic breathing or progressive muscle relaxation to prepare for sleep. These practices activate the vagus nerve and help lower cortisol levels, which can promote deeper, more restorative sleep.
- **Avoid Stimulating Activities:** Try to reduce exposure to screens and other distractions in the hour or so before bed. This allows your nervous system to enter a more relaxed state, supporting the natural release of melatonin for sleep.

Success Stories: Real-Life Examples of Vagus Mastery

Case Study 1: Overcoming Chronic Stress with Deep Breathing

Sarah, a corporate executive, struggled with high levels of stress, particularly before important meetings. She frequently found herself feeling overwhelmed and anxious, which negatively affected her performance and health. After learning about the vagus nerve and its connection to stress regulation, she began practicing deep breathing exercises daily. Specifically, she focused on slow, deep inhales through her nose, followed by long exhales through her mouth.

After a few weeks of consistent practice, Sarah noticed a significant improvement in her ability to remain calm and focused during stressful situations. She also began integrating deep breathing into her morning routine, and as a result, felt more energized and emotionally balanced throughout the day. She attributed this shift to the increased activation of her vagus nerve, which helped her manage stress and enhance her emotional resilience.

Case Study 2: Improving Mental Clarity with Meditation

David, a college student, often struggled with brain fog, lack of focus, and mental fatigue, particularly during exam periods. Despite his best efforts, his inability to concentrate was affecting his academic performance. A friend recommended he try meditation as a way to enhance cognitive function and reduce stress. David committed to a daily practice of mindfulness meditation, combined with diaphragmatic breathing.

After a few weeks, David experienced a notable improvement in both his mental clarity and stress levels. The vagus nerve stimulation through meditation helped calm his nervous system, reducing the anxiety that often accompanied studying and exam preparation. He reported feeling more present and less distracted during his study sessions, which translated into improved performance.

Case Study 3: Healing Gut Health through Vagal Stimulation

Maria, a 40-year-old woman, had long struggled with digestive issues, including bloating, constipation, and irregular bowel movements. After seeing numerous specialists with little success, she decided to explore holistic methods for gut health. She came across the connection between the vagus nerve and the gut-brain axis and began incorporating vagus nerve-stimulating practices such as slow, deep breathing and mindfulness meditation into her routine.

Within a few weeks of consistent practice, Maria noticed significant improvements in her digestion. Her bloating decreased, and her bowel movements became more regular. She believes that by strengthening her vagal tone and activating the parasympathetic nervous system, she was able to better regulate her gut function and overall well-being.

Creating a Personalized Plan for Vagal Wellness

Mastering the vagus nerve requires a tailored approach that aligns with your lifestyle, goals, and challenges. Here's how you can create a personalized plan to enhance your vagal health:

1. Identify Your Vagal Health Goals

Reflect on your specific health concerns and how they might be influenced by vagal tone. Are you looking to reduce stress, improve sleep, enhance cognitive function, or address digestive issues? Write down your goals and focus on the areas where you most need improvement.

2. Choose Your Vagal Stimulation Techniques

- Based on your goals, choose a combination of vagal stimulation practices that resonate with you. You might focus on deep breathing for stress relief, meditation for emotional regulation, or cold exposure to increase alertness and energy.
- Aim to practice at least one vagus nerve technique each day, whether it's through breathing exercises, meditation, or incorporating physical movement.

3. Integrate Practices into Your Routine

Integrating vagus nerve activation into your daily routine is crucial for long-term benefits. Whether it's a morning breathing ritual, mindful movement during breaks, or evening meditation before bed, choose practices that are easy to incorporate into your life.

4. Track Your Progress

Monitor how you feel as you implement these practices. Are you feeling less stressed, more focused, or experiencing better digestion? Keep a journal of your progress, noting any improvements or setbacks. This will help you fine-tune your plan as you go along.

5. Make Adjustments as Needed

As you begin to master vagus nerve techniques, adjust your plan based on your experiences. You may find that you want to add more techniques or refine your focus on particular areas. The goal is to make these practices a sustainable part of your lifestyle.

Conclusion

Mastering the vagus nerve and integrating its benefits into daily life is a powerful way to enhance your physical, mental, and emotional health. The real-world applications of vagus nerve techniques can lead to profound transformation, from reducing stress and improving cognitive function to healing the gut and fostering emotional regulation. By taking a proactive approach to vagal wellness and incorporating simple, effective practices into your routine, you can unlock the full potential of your body's silent master and create lasting positive change.

Chapter 25: Mastering the Vagus Nerve for a Thriving Life

The journey to mastering the vagus nerve is one of empowerment, resilience, and holistic well-being. This final chapter brings together all of the insights and practical techniques shared throughout the book, guiding you on how to integrate them into a thriving, long-term health plan. Mastering the vagus nerve is not a one-time event but a continuous process of tuning into your body, mind, and emotions. By consistently practicing the principles in this book, you can experience improved physical health, emotional balance, and mental clarity.

In this chapter, we will summarize the key takeaways from the entire book, explore how to maintain long-term health through vagal activation, and provide guidance on how to continue your journey of vagus nerve mastery in the years to come.

Key Takeaways from Mastering the Vagus Nerve

The vagus nerve is one of the most important and powerful components of the human body. Its far-reaching influence on various systems makes it a central player in health, emotional regulation, and overall well-being. By mastering the vagus nerve, you unlock the ability to:

1. **Regulate Stress and Anxiety**: Through practices like deep breathing, mindfulness, and meditation, you can activate the parasympathetic nervous system, reducing the harmful effects of chronic stress and anxiety. This empowers you to navigate the challenges of life with greater emotional resilience.
2. **Enhance Physical Health**: From improving heart rate variability to boosting immunity, vagal stimulation has profound effects on your physical health. Incorporating regular exercise, proper nutrition, and sleep rituals helps promote vagal tone and optimize your body's natural healing processes.
3. **Improve Mental and Emotional Well-Being**: Strengthening the vagus nerve contributes to improved mood, mental clarity, and emotional stability. The vagus nerve plays a key role in balancing neurotransmitters like serotonin and dopamine, which directly impact mental health.
4. **Promote Gut Health**: The gut-brain axis is another area where the vagus nerve plays a significant role. By enhancing vagal tone, you can improve digestion, regulate the gut microbiome, and reduce symptoms of gastrointestinal disorders like bloating, constipation, and irritable bowel syndrome (IBS).
5. **Support Long-Term Aging and Resilience**: As you age, maintaining high vagal tone is essential for reducing inflammation and preventing age-related diseases. The vagus nerve is involved in immune regulation, and strengthening it helps protect against chronic conditions, promoting longevity and quality of life.

How to Maintain Long-Term Health Through Vagal Activation

Mastery of the vagus nerve is not something that happens overnight—it is a lifelong process of developing habits that promote balance and health. To continue experiencing the benefits of vagal stimulation, it's essential to incorporate these practices into your daily routine and lifestyle. Here are some strategies to maintain long-term vagal health:

1. Consistent Vagus Nerve Stimulation

Regular practices such as deep breathing, diaphragmatic breathing, and mindfulness meditation should become part of your everyday routine. Even a few minutes a day can have a lasting impact on your overall health and emotional well-being.

2. Balanced Diet and Gut Health

Focus on eating a nutrient-dense diet rich in anti-inflammatory foods. Foods like omega-3 fatty acids, fiber, and fermented foods help support gut health and reduce inflammation, promoting healthy vagal function.

3. Regular Physical Activity

Continue engaging in activities that promote vagal tone, such as yoga, aerobic exercise, and walking. These not only help activate the vagus nerve but also boost your mood, reduce stress, and improve cardiovascular health.

4. Prioritize Sleep and Recovery

Ensure you are getting enough restorative sleep each night. Poor sleep reduces vagal tone, while quality sleep enhances the parasympathetic response and supports overall health. Consider incorporating relaxation techniques like progressive muscle relaxation or listening to calming music before bed.

5. Build Emotional Resilience

Use mindfulness and emotional regulation techniques to handle negative emotions. Emotional regulation is key to vagal health, as chronic stress can diminish vagal tone. By developing greater emotional intelligence, you can enhance your ability to stay calm and centered, even in difficult situations.

Continuing the Journey: Living with Vagal Mastery

Mastering the vagus nerve is an ongoing journey of self-discovery and improvement. Here's how you can continue this process and make it a permanent part of your life:

1. Reflect and Adjust Regularly

Take time each week to reflect on your health and well-being. How are you feeling emotionally and physically? Are there areas where you could focus more on strengthening your vagal tone? Be open to adjusting your practices based on your current needs.

2. Seek Support and Community

Surround yourself with like-minded individuals who are also focused on wellness and personal growth. Whether it's through online groups, local meetups, or health seminars, sharing your experiences and learning from others can help you stay motivated and inspired.

3. Embrace New Technologies and Techniques

Stay informed about emerging technologies and new research on vagus nerve stimulation. Wearables, biohacking techniques, and advanced vagus nerve stimulation tools may offer new ways to enhance your health and well-being.

4. Celebrate Progress

Acknowledge the positive changes you experience as a result of your efforts. Whether it's a reduction in stress, improved sleep, or better gut health, celebrating your successes reinforces your commitment to maintaining a healthy vagus nerve.

Conclusion

Mastering the vagus nerve is one of the most empowering things you can do for your health and happiness. By harnessing the power of the vagus nerve, you unlock the ability to regulate stress, enhance emotional well-being, improve physical health, and foster resilience. The practices shared in this book are not just tools; they are life-changing habits that, when applied consistently, can transform every aspect of your life.

As you continue to implement the techniques and principles outlined in this book, remember that the journey to vagal mastery is ongoing. Your vagus nerve is a powerful ally, and by nurturing it, you are setting the stage for a lifetime of health, happiness, and balance.

Embrace the change. Transform your life with vagal mastery and step into a future where your health and well-being are in your hands.

The future of vagus nerve research is bright, and new discoveries will continue to shape our understanding of how to optimize this vital pathway. As the science evolves, so too will the practices that can help you thrive. The journey is just beginning.

www.ingramcontent.com/pod-product-compliance
Lightning Source LLC
Chambersburg PA
CBHW082248220526
45469CB00009B/2920